RENAISSANCE SURGEONS

This book examines the lives, careers, and publications of a group of Spanish Renaissance surgeons as exemplars of both the surgical renaissance occurring across Europe and of the unique context of Spain.

In the sixteenth century, European surgeons forged new identities as learned experts who combined university medical degrees with manual skills and practical experience. No longer merely apprentice-trained craftsmen engaged only with healing the exterior wounds and rashes of the body, these learned surgeons actively engaged with the epistemic shifts of the sixteenth century, including new forms of knowledge construction, based in empiricism, and knowledge circulation, based in printing. These surgeons have long been overshadowed by the innovative work of anatomists and botanists but were participants in the same intellectual currents reshaping many aspects of knowledge. Active in communities across both Castile and Aragon, learned surgeons formed an intellectual community of practitioners and scholars who helped reshape surgical knowledge and practice. This book provides an overview of the Spanish learned surgeons, known as *médicos y cirujanos*, who were influential in universities, on battlefields, at court, and in private practice. It argues that the surgeons' larger significance rests in their collective identity as part of the broader intellectual shift to empiricism and innovation of the Renaissance.

Renaissance Surgeons: Learning and Expertise in the Age of Print is essential reading for upper-level students and scholars of the history of medicine and early modern Spain.

Kristy Wilson Bowers is Assistant Professor of History at the University of Missouri. She is the author of *Plague and Public Health in Early Modern Seville* (2013), as well as several articles related to the history of medicine in early modern Spain.

The Body in the City

This series aims to intersect and to energise two strands in historical studies: the pre-modern city as an historical subject (encompassing political institutions, rituals, built environments, religious activities, etc) and histories of the premodern body with their debates about how bodies are shaped by discourse and context. The series will highlight approaches which emphasize the vernacular as revealed by new sources and novel approaches to them. While there are numerous studies of the body in history, this series will explore critically and in innovative ways the relationship between bodies and environments. This will allow scholars involved to analyse how particular spaces, locations and physical *milieux* affect understandings of the body and govern responses to particular problems. The multi-disciplinary approach to the topic places the series at the leading edge of its field.
Series Editors: Peter Howard, *Monash University, Australia*, and John Henderson, *University of Cambridge, UK.*

In this series:

Gaspare Tagliacozzi and Early Modern Surgery
Faces, Men, and Pain
Paolo Savoia

Popular Politics in an Aristocratic Republic
Political Conflict and Social Contestation in Late Medieval and Early Modern Venice
Edited by Maartje Van Gelder and Claire Judde De Larivière

Representing Infirmity
Diseased Bodies in Renaissance Italy
Edited by John Henderson, Fredrika Jacobs and Jonathan K. Nelson

Renaissance Surgeons
Learning and Expertise in the Age of Print
Kristy Wilson Bowers

For more information about this series, please visit: https://www.routledge.com/The-Body-in-the-City/book-series/BOCY

RENAISSANCE SURGEONS

Learning and Expertise in the Age of Print

Kristy Wilson Bowers

Routledge
Taylor & Francis Group
LONDON AND NEW YORK

Cover image: Science History Images/Alamy Stock Photo

First published 2023
by Routledge
4 Park Square, Milton Park, Abingdon, Oxon OX14 4RN

and by Routledge
605 Third Avenue, New York, NY 10158

Routledge is an imprint of the Taylor & Francis Group, an informa business

British Library Cataloguing-in-Publication Data
A catalogue record for this book is available from the British Library

Library of Congress Cataloging-in-Publication Data
Names: Bowers, Kristy Wilson, author.
Title: Renaissance surgeons : learning and expertise in the age of print / Kristy Wilson Bowers.
Description: Abingdon, Oxon ; New York, NY : Routledge, 2023. | Series: The body in the city | Includes bibliographical references and index.
Identifiers: LCCN 2022023082 (print) | LCCN 2022023083 (ebook) | ISBN 9781032270401 (hardback) | ISBN 9781032270418 (paperback) | ISBN 9781003291060 (ebook)
Subjects: LCSH: Surgery--Study and teaching--Spain--History--16th century. | Surgery--Study and teaching--Spain--History--17th century. | Surgery--Spain--History--16th century. | Surgery--Spain--History--17th century. | Surgeons--Spain--History--16th century. | Surgeons--Spain--History--17th century.
Classification: LCC RD28.S7 B69 2023 (print) | LCC RD28.S7 (ebook) | DDC 617.0076--dc23/eng/20220713
LC record available at https://lccn.loc.gov/2022023082
LC ebook record available at https://lccn.loc.gov/2022023083

ISBN: 978-1-032-27040-1 (hbk)
ISBN: 978-1-032-27041-8 (pbk)
ISBN: 978-1-003-29106-0 (ebk)

DOI: 10.4324/9781003291060

Typeset in Bembo
by SPi Technologies India Pvt Ltd (Straive)

In memory of Helen Nader, an inspirational scholar and mentor

CONTENTS

List of Figures ix
Preface and Acknowledgments x

Introduction 1

1 Physicians and Surgeons: Medical Learning and Licensing 13
Ancient and Medieval Surgery 13
Medieval Education 14
Medical Humanism 16
Regulating Medicine 19
Regulating Education in Spain 21
The Médico y Cirujano 23

2 Spanish Learned Surgeons: A Broad and Connected Movement 30
Royal Service 33
Court Surgeons 33
Military Surgeons 37
Teaching and Practicing: Universities and Hospitals 39
Print Networks 46
Citing Each Other 46
Referencing Others 48

3 Sharing Knowledge: Learned Surgical Texts 56
Foundations 56
Language and Authority 58
Print Culture 63

4 Refining Knowledge and Practice: Empiricism, Tradition, and Innovation 72
Medicine and Empiricism 75
Refining Knowledge and Practice 80
Refining Wound Treatment 81
Revisiting and Refining Trepanation 86

5 Expanding Surgical Expertise: Addressing New Problems 100
Urology 101
Legal and Forensic Medicine 105
Gunpowder Wounds 107
New Diseases 110
Typhus and Plague 111
Morbo Gálico or the Great Pox 113

Conclusion 121

Appendix: Brief Biographies of Spanish Learned Surgeons 125
Bibliography 132
Index 155

FIGURES

0.1 Map of Spain 6
2.1 Portrait of Bartolomé Hidalgo de Agüero, from Francisco Pacheco, *Book of Portraits of Illustrious and Memorable Men* (1599) 45
3.1 The first page of the *Avisos Particulares* as reprinted in Bartolomé Hidalgo de Agüero, *Tesoro de la verdadera cirugía* (1604) 65
4.1 Illustration of head wounds from Andrés Alcázar, *Chirurgiae libri sex* (1575) 87
4.2 Illustration of the handle and points of a trepans from Andrés Alcázar, *Chirurgiae libri sex* (1575) 92
5.1 Title page from Francisco Díaz, *Tratado nuevamente impresso de todas las enfermedades de los riñones, vexiga, y carnosidades de la verga, y urina* (1588) 103
5.2 Illustration of a tool developed by Francisco Díaz to treat urethral stricture. Francisco Díaz, *Tratado nuevamente impresso de todas las enfermedades de los riñones, vexiga, y carnosidades de la verga, y urina* (1588) 105

PREFACE AND ACKNOWLEDGMENTS

This book grew out of research that began decades ago in Seville when I was working on plague epidemics and the public health response to them. In the midst of city council records, I came across one of these surgeons, Bartolomé Hidalgo de Agüero. He was embroiled in a dispute with another surgeon over a broadsheet he had published (*Avisos Particulares*), and the men had each given written accounts of their arguments for and against particular forms of treatment. The city archive seemed an odd place to find a dispute over medical practices, but it was an intriguing exchange, and I mentally filed it away for later. It took a decade until I eventually returned to it and wrote an article about him. The research for that article led me to several other surgeons, including Hidalgo de Agüero's greatest opponent, Juan Fragoso. In the intervening years, as I completed other projects, Hidalgo de Agüero and his fellow surgeons stayed with me, eventually becoming the focus of this book.

As I read more deeply in the Spanish historical literature, many of the same names kept arising, cited by scholars as important, influential, and innovative surgeons: Juan Calvo, Juan Fragoso, Bartolomé Hidalgo de Agüero, Francisco Díaz, Dionisio Daza Chacón. Juan Fragoso, in fact, turned out to be the linking thread of a conference panel at the Association for Spanish and Portuguese Historical Studies in 2016, though we had not realized it beforehand. I referred to his work as a surgeon in my presentation on learned surgeons, while Paula De Vos referred to his work on medical botany in her presentation on transatlantic pharmacology, and Luis Corteguera referred to him as court physician-surgeon in his presentation on Spanish views of monarchy, referring to his views on the healing power known as the "royal touch." This struck me as an apt encapsulation of the broad intellectual reach of many learned surgeons. While I began with surgeons who wrote in the vernacular, I realized that I needed to expand to include two men who wrote in Latin, Andrés Alcázar and Francisco Arceo, who were also active in the same decades and whose texts were very influential. Rounding out the group are two slightly lesser-known figures, Andrés de León and Antonio Pérez, who I realized not only fit the parameters I had set but also were surprisingly connected to Dionisio Daza Chacón. Certainly, there are many others who could be included in a study of Renaissance learned surgeons, but these nine nicely reflect the diversity and influence of learned surgeons.

A project this long in the making owes an enormous debt to many institutions and colleagues—too many to name. I first offer my thanks and acknowledgment to the many Spanish historians of medicine who have been writing about these learned surgeons for decades. There is a long and rich tradition of the history of medicine in Spain, particularly in the medieval and early modern eras. Historians there have done significant work pulling information from the archives and writing inciteful analyses. Their names appear throughout the notes and bibliography, but I feel a need to point to them collectively at the outset. This work could not have been written without them. The Biblioteca Nacional in Madrid; National Library of Medicine in Bethesda, Maryland; and Biblioteca de la Universidad de Sevilla provided access to many texts of the sixteenth (and later) centuries. In addition, I thank librarians at both Northern Illinois University where I started this project and the University of Missouri where I finished it, who have helped me track down many foreign works. To the same end, I am also immensely grateful for recent efforts of digitization and open access publishing, particularly within Spain, which has also considerably enhanced access to many resources, both primary and secondary.

Friends, acquaintances, and strangers have listened and responded to pieces of this book at conferences of the Association for Spanish and Portuguese Historical Studies, the American Association for the History of Medicine, Sixteenth Century Studies, the Renaissance Society of America, the Southern Association for the History of Medicine and Science, Scientiae, and the Premodern Spanish Historical Association of the Midwest. Those venues provided stimulating atmospheres that sparked helpful conversations not only related to this project but about research in general. Special thanks to Grace Coolidge and Valentina Tikoff for their enduring support over the years, as well as to Ann Carmichael, Dan Crews, Michelle Clouse, Luis Corteguera, Sylvia Mitchell, Gretchen Starr-LeBeau, Liz Lehfeldt, Scott Taylor, Pam Beattie, Miriam Shadis, Jeff Bowman, and Daniel Wasserman-Soler for feedback and helpful conversations. Thanks as well to the series editors, Peter Howard and John Henderson, as well as everyone at Routledge for making the publication process so smooth.

Finally, heartfelt thanks to the family who helped provide me with time to work on this: to the Wilsons for always being the support hub and staging center; to the Filbeys for hosting meals, providing so much transportation, and always having great stories to share; to the Bowers for leaving a light on and having a bed ready; to the Cupps for flexibility and understanding and most of all to J. D., Caroline, and Julia for their constant support, patience, and love.

INTRODUCTION

The sixteenth century was an era of change across nearly all aspects of European life. As evocatively described by Porter and Teich, this era was the culmination of "the new culture, the new religion, the new economic formations, the New World, and, not least, the new science."[1] The new science of this era included medicine, which underwent challenges to both theory and practice, as well as an expansion in pharmacopoeia, with new attention to *materia medica* (both from the New World and found locally in Europe) and a revolution in anatomical studies.[2] Surgery also changed during this era, as increasing numbers of university-educated surgeons emerged in the courts and on the battlefields, offering new forms of expertise and publishing texts that both solidified and expanded their field.

Surgery has been often overlooked as a medical field for the sixteenth and seventeenth centuries. Scholars have paid attention to a handful of prominent individuals, such as Giovanni da Vigo and Ambroise Paré, both of whom published influential texts that were translated into many languages. But unlike earlier centuries, for which medieval scholars have long provided rich and layered analyses, much remains unknown about the contours of surgical education and practice in the early modern era. In the last decade, however, an increasing number of scholars have begun this work, offering new insights on individuals and practices, illuminating both the standards and changes of early modern surgery, particularly "the shifting boundaries between surgery and physic and the relationship between theory, practice, and skills."[3]

That boundary, of physic and surgery, was indeed a moving target. The most common boundary recognized by scholars has been that of practice: early modern physicians were largely hands-off and treated the internal, while surgeons were hands-on and treated the external (and often messier) problems of the body—wounds, abscesses, rashes, and so forth. In addition, we find a second boundary of education: physicians were distinguished as having knowledge of theory, gained

DOI: 10.4324/9781003291060-1

from books studied at universities. Surgeons, on the other hand, we are often told, were apprentice-trained in skills and practices. But we know that many practitioners crossed those boundaries of both learning and the body itself: surgeons were often literate and sometimes held university degrees; physicians engaged in (and gained fame for) the hands-on process of dissection that made them anatomists. While thirteenth-century surgical authors, who were clearly knowledgeable and wrote in Latin, such as Guglielmo of Saliceto (d. 1277) and Lanfranc of Milan (d. 1306?), are clearly identified as surgeons, some surgical writers in the next century, such as Dino del Garbo (d. 1327) and Guy de Chauliac (d. 1368), are identified as physicians.[4]

By the sixteenth century, those lines become even blurrier as the same person could act (and be identified) as various combinations of physician, surgeon, anatomist, botanist, and apothecary. Anatomists and botanists, even if principally engaged in teaching and publishing on these fields, were trained in medicine, though whether they held the position/title of physician or surgeon varied. Berengario da Carpi is the rare well-known anatomist who clearly identified himself as a practicing surgeon. Gabriele Falloppio was a physician and anatomist, who also held university chairs in surgery and botany. The Czech physician Jan Jessen, rector of the University of Wittenberg, was also "professor of anatomy, surgery, and botany, and author of a series of texts on anatomy, surgery, and natural philosophy."[5] Perhaps the most famous anatomist, Andreas Vesalius, was a physician appointed to the chair of surgery at Padua, from which he revolutionized the study of anatomy. He is rarely identified as a surgeon, though he did later act as one on the battlefield after entering Imperial service with Charles V. Among Vesalius's students were Pedro Jimeno and Luis Collado, both of whom later held a variety of medical professorships at the University of Valencia, teaching courses in anatomy, as well as medicine and surgery. It becomes increasingly difficult to determine who to label a surgeon in the sixteenth century, or how useful such labels even are.

Despite this blurring of boundaries, however, surgery still retained a separate identity. In part, the separation of labels for physician and surgeon endures because what appears most often in the historical records are moments of dispute—in particular when elite physicians sought to assert superiority and authority over other medical practitioners—which tend to leave evidence more readily than moments of peaceful coexistence. These disputes can give us a false sense of separation and contention between medical disciplines. Yet just as often, distinctions did remain, and separate titles continued to be used in many contexts. In his study of medical teaching in sixteenth-century Padua, particularly of the men who taught surgery, Bylebyl notes, "It is a nice question whether such individuals should be considered as physicians who practiced surgery or as surgeons who had taken medical degrees, but the fact is that while they were free to practice internal medicine, they functioned essentially as the elite of surgical practitioners and teachers, and were often referred to as 'surgeons.'"[6] Surgical practice remained grounded in skilled technique, even when contextualized by medical theory. Outside of universities, surgeons in some places might belong to a college or guild (of surgeons or of barber-surgeons), though members of surgical guilds did not necessarily practice surgery.[7]

In the Renaissance, there existed a wide range of practitioners who identified as surgeons, from barber-surgeon to physician-surgeon, apprentice-trained to university-educated. In general, it is the educational boundary that seems to hold most firm—those with university degrees were most often considered physicians. Surgeon remained a lesser title, to be carefully raised in status by noting "learned" if the individual in question had a university degree. Likewise, learned men who published texts are often assumed to be physicians, even if they practiced surgery, or are often labeled anatomists if that is what they published on. Skaarup in his text on Spanish Renaissance anatomists refers to "the renowned anatomist and urologist Francisco Díaz" as well as "[a]nother anatomist, Juan Fragoso."[8] Both men certainly included anatomy in their texts, as do many other surgeons of their era, but neither is known for conducting anatomical dissections nor for teaching anatomy. Rather, they identified themselves with the title of *médico y cirujano* (doctor and surgeon), which emphasized both their learned status and their surgical practice. This dual title became common in sixteenth-century Spain, and similar titles can be found among practitioners in other countries as well. In itself, this dual title may be seen to reinforce the separation between physic and surgery as opposed to uniting the two fields. However, it is clear that the Spanish médicos y cirujanos, who are the focus of this study, were working to promote surgery as a profession both skilled and learned.

Multiple factors helped increase the prominence and status of surgery as a discipline, as well as of individual surgeons, in this era. Above all was the increased demand for surgeons to treat the wounds, fractures, dislocations, and epidemics that resulted from increased warfare (including wounds from both swords and gunpowder weapons), voyages of exploration and colonization, local upheavals of protests and rebellions, and the ever-erupting epidemic diseases, including plague, syphilis, and typhus. With increased demand came increased experience for the men who could treat all manner of wounds and diseases, especially under the challenging conditions on battlefields, onboard ships, and in exploratory expeditions. In addition, the expansion of Spanish colonial territories brought increased demand for learned surgical texts that could help train or improve the practices of colonial surgeons. Yet Renaissance surgeons were not only immersed in the active life of battle and exploration; they were also immersed in the intellectual world of humanist study and teaching.

Alongside this increased need for surgeons came two other changes that proved important for sixteenth-century surgeons—the acceptance of the vernacular as a learned/scientific language and the continued expansion of printing, both of which had significant roots in the previous century. Thus, the convergence of political, social, economic, and intellectual trends helped bring about a renaissance of surgery, one accessible through printed texts, often in the vernacular, which exploded in number throughout the century across Europe.[9] These texts are particularly important for understanding early modern surgery, as surgeons left few other records. The French surgeon Ambroise Paré published many treatises at mid-century, helping to cement his reputation then and now as an innovative and successful surgeon. He is most often cited today as the "father of modern surgery," though he was very much a product of his time, working on many of the same ideas as others. He simply published earlier and more accessibly. The seventeenth-century English surgeon Joseph Binns, whose casebooks have been studied by Lucinda McCray Beier, is an exception, as are the casebooks of medical astrologers Simon Forman and Richard Napier, studied by Lauren Kassell.[10] Records of practice are somewhat more available for physicians, who wrote in a variety of genres, including, from the late sixteenth century on, collected case studies known as *observationes*.[11] Most surgeons, however, left fewer traces of their lives and careers. The personal information we have about them is mostly what they chose to include in their texts. Other information about them can be pieced together from official sources—royal court records, institutional records such as from universities and hospitals where they studied or worked, municipal records, and parish records that have yielded some personal details such as marriages, births, and deaths, and petitions for payment for services rendered. While they did not produce personal diaries or casebooks, the Spanish surgeons studied here did include both illustrative case studies and personal anecdotes within their larger surgical manuals.

The center of this study is a generation of innovative university-educated physician-surgeons who practiced, taught, and wrote in sixteenth-century Spain. Well-known to historians of medicine within Spain, they have received scant attention elsewhere.[12] While earlier generations of historians who wrote about them tended to do so in the vein of "great men," this study seeks to place them back within their context—they were both derivative and innovative, both insular and international in outlook and reputation, both influential on and influenced by what their peers were doing across Europe. In many ways, as we will see, their work was directly parallel to what was happening across other parts of Europe. In other ways, however, they were uniquely innovative in developing and advocating for new techniques and concepts. While the republic of medical letters to which they belonged was an international one, the politics of learning, licensing, and practicing medicine were always local and differed across different geographies. Thus, although these Spanish authors frequently cite the work of many contemporaries, they practiced and formed their ideas in a uniquely Spanish context, one that had contours often quite different from the French, English, Italian or German ones. Like many of their counterparts in other nations, they sought new knowledge and new ways of sharing knowledge, pushing back against the notion of surgeons as akin to mere "unskilled" or "unlettered" barbers. In their interactions with one another, including the debates they carried out among themselves, in the empiricism and innovative spirit they showed, and in their efforts to redefine what surgery encompassed, they mirrored what was happening across Western Europe.

Renaissance Spain

Spanish learned surgeons were educated and practiced in an era of change for the Iberian Peninsula. "Renaissance" can be a frustratingly vague term, used to refer to a general era in history (which can be anywhere from the fourteenth to the seventeenth century), an intellectual movement, known as humanism (the revival of ancient written sources, along with new linguistics and literary forms, new modes of critical thinking and the spread of new ideas via movable type printing), and an artistic movement (associated with new uses of perspective, secularism, and the recognition of individual talent). In this study, it is used as a shorthand to encompass both a time period (the late fifteenth through the sixteenth centuries) and a series of linked intellectual shifts: an interest in new translations or editions of ancient authors coupled with an increasing critical assessment of that learning, an embrace of experience and experiment as valid new sources of learning, the increased use of vernacular languages by learned men alongside Latin, and the use of printing to disseminate these ideas to a broader audience than ever before.

In Spanish historiography, the Renaissance is most often linked to the rule of Fernando and Isabel, whose 1469 marriage brought the crowns of Castile and Aragon into joint rule, laying the groundwork for unification of the territories into Spain. It also enabled the pooling of resources, both manpower and financial, for the final defeat of the remnant Muslim territory of the Emirate of Granada in 1492. Despite the successes of unification, however, the political, economic, and cultural distinctions between Castile and Aragon remained intact for centuries, until the eighteenth-century reforms of the Bourbon Dynasty. Even within each of these territories, regionalism abounded. The centuries-long processes of conquest, marriage, and inheritance by which these territories had been consolidated into large kingdoms meant that they remained fractured in many ways. The divisions of religion and politics were compounded by geography and climate, resulting in distinct cultures. Galicia in northwestern Iberia remained quite different from Andalucía in the south, despite both being in the Kingdom of Castile. More entrenched fragmentation existed in the Crown of Aragon, which was composed of the separate territories of the Kingdom of Aragon, the Kingdom of Valencia, and the Principality of Catalonia (see Figure 0.1). After 1512, the Kingdom of Navarre was added to Aragonese control as well. Though recognizing a common ruler, each of these states retained distinct political and judicial systems along with distinct cultural (and linguistic) traditions. The joint reign of Fernando and Isabel marks an important turning point, then, in laying the groundwork for consolidation of power across these disparate territories but did not usher in true unity. This political consolidation did, however, lead to a new intellectual flourishing that resulted from an era of relative peace and stability.

Political entanglements between the Crown of Aragon and southern Italian territories, dating to the thirteenth century, resulted in ongoing cultural and intellectual exchanges, bringing a flow of intellectual crosscurrents from Italy and other parts of Europe. The work of early Italian humanists, including Petrarch (1304–74) and Boccaccio (1313–75), reached Aragonese courts in the late fourteenth century, sparking an early interest there in Latin linguistics.[13] Fourteenth- and fifteenth-century rulers in both Castile and Aragon were at times significant patrons of arts and letters, particularly after the mid-fifteenth century. Italian humanist chroniclers at the Trastámara court of Isabel and Fernando may have overemphasized the

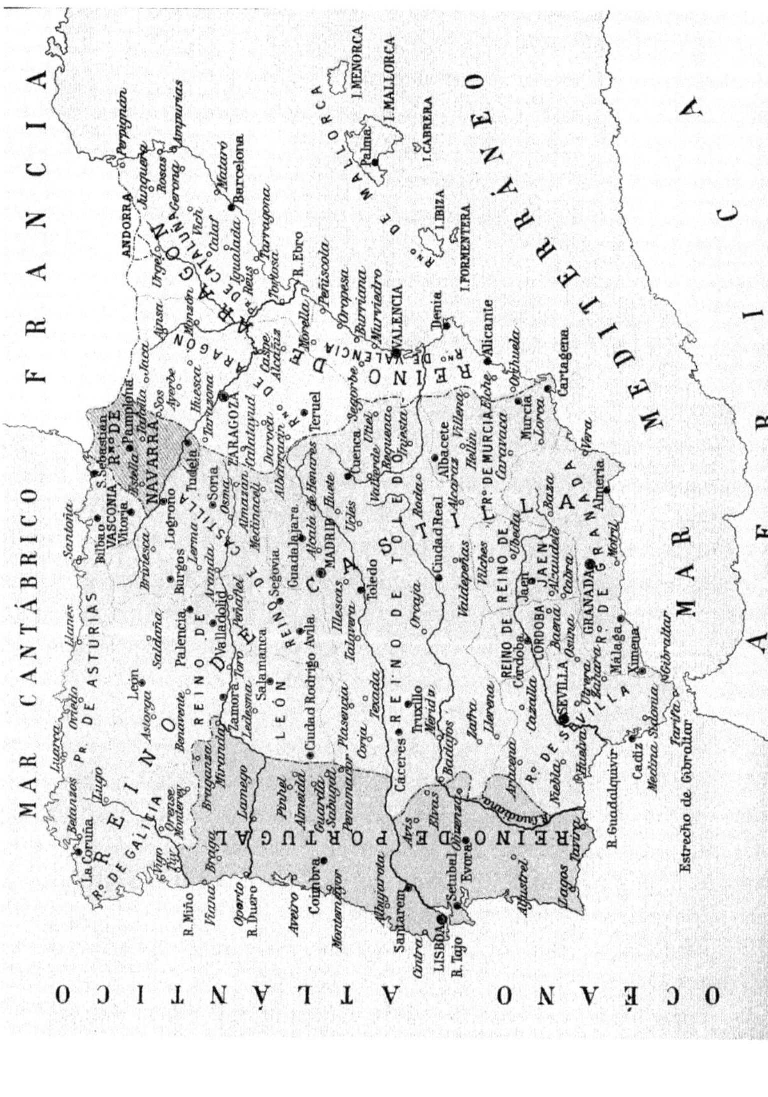

FIGURE 0.1 Map of Spain (Alamy Stock Photo).

role of the Catholic monarchs and underemphasized earlier patrons in bringing Renaissance thought to Iberia, but it is certainly true that the union of the crowns enabled a more consistent flourishing of patronage of arts, language, and textual studies.[14] Best known of the Spanish humanists of this era was Antonio de Nebrija (1444–1522), an important intellectual (and tireless self-promoter), who produced influential works on Latin and Spanish grammar, including the earliest work of Spanish grammar and an early Spanish dictionary.[15] The entanglements and influences between Spain and Italy continued and expanded in the next century during the reigns of both Charles V and Philip II, whose ties to various Italian city-states were reinforced through diplomacy, wars, patronage, and charity.[16]

These Spanish Renaissance trends of the consolidation of royal power and the embrace of humanism are also evident when we turn to examine the history of medicine and surgery. The consolidation of royal power included its extension into the foundation and patronage of new universities as well as royal intervention in medical education and licensing in the name of public health. Humanism gave new impetus to the translation of ancient texts, the expanded use of the vernacular (both Catalan and Castilian) for scientific and medical texts, and the production and publication of new learned texts. This laid the groundwork for the resurgence of learned surgery in Spain from its late medieval roots.

Spanish Learned Surgeons

The learned surgeons who are the focus of this study are well-known in Spanish literature on the history of medicine. Luis Granjel, a foundational figure in the history of medicine in Spain, and graduate students working under him, carried out an incredible amount of primary research to bring to light the work of these surgeons, as well as many other medical figures. In addition to his own work, he established the *Seminario de historia de la medicina* at the University of Salamanca in the 1950s, publishing through the university press a series of short monographs analyzing the publications of many Spanish medical authors. In subsequent decades, the University of Valencia emerged as another key center for the study of the history of medicine, founded and led by José María López Piñero. More recent scholars, such as José Fresquet Febrero, Pedro Conde Parrado, Joaquín Herrera Dávila, María Luz López Terrada, and many others have continued to refine our understanding of learned surgeons and their work.[17] Unfortunately, and rather inexplicably, this work has not received the attention it should have outside of Spain, particularly in English language scholarship.

This study focuses on a group of elite and highly educated *cirujanos latinos*. The title they most often used, médico y cirujano, demonstrated their medical education and surgical skills. Therefore, this study most often uses the term "learned surgeon" in referring to them. The core set of learned surgeons who are at the heart of this study were nine men: Andrés Alcázar (c.1490–c.1585), Francisco Arceo (1493–1580), Dionisio Daza Chacón (1503 or 1510–96), Juan Fragoso (1530–97), Bartolomé Hidalgo de Agüero (1531–97), Francisco Díaz (c. 1530–90), Juan Calvo

(1535–99), Antonio Pérez (fl. 1567–1604), and Andrés de León (fl. 1568–1605). There were quite a few other Spanish surgeons (and even more physicians) who published treatises in the sixteenth century, but I have chosen to focus specifically on these nine based on several criteria. First, they were surgeons who gained university degrees in medicine before surgery courses were offered in any Spanish universities but who chose to also learn and practice surgery. Second, they all published treatises on surgery (and some on other related medical topics) that in some way changed or expanded surgical knowledge. They were key innovators whose use of experience and observation led them to improve various surgical methods and to develop new surgical instruments. They expanded the surgeon's expertise not only in education and training but also in what conditions fell under the purview of surgery.

The men included in this study formed a collective with varying ties connecting them into a loose network. Though some were friends and colleagues, others knew each other only through reputation or the texts they published. We may think of them as connected in a series of interlocking circles, whose variables included geographic proximity, temporal overlap at one of Spain's universities offering medical training, mutual interests, courtly and military networks, publishing houses, and even intermediary third parties. They merit a book focused on them, both as individuals and as a collective group, because they were influential in their own times and for at least a century beyond. In the work they did and the texts they produced, they embody the larger intellectual changes at work across Europe in the sixteenth century—the rise of empiricism, the expanded use of the printing press, the push for new professional status and respect, the response to new diseases. They were intellectuals and innovators who witnessed key events of the sixteenth century and whose students and texts carried their influence through the next century and in some cases even beyond. Indeed, their reputations continue today as key Renaissance innovators. [18] What makes them more striking is that though they were born in different decades, some as early as 1490 and others not until the mid-1530s, they published in the same era, roughly between 1560 and 1605. Most did not live into the next century, dying between 1585 and 1599, perhaps excepting the two youngest, Pérez and León, whose deaths are known only as to have been after their final publications in 1598 and 1605, respectively.

Perhaps most significantly, these surgeons were all university educated and then chose to practice surgery, a profession that, at the time they started their careers, did not require university training. Most of them went on to achieve high positions at court or universities. They offered their treatises as active surgeons who genuinely sought to expand and elevate treatment, knowledge, and perhaps to elevate the reputation of surgeons. All of the surgeons discussed in this book authored at least two volumes, most of them one on surgery and one on a related topic such as anatomy, disease, or materia medica (see appendix). To take just the five best-known authors (Juan Calvo, Dionisio Daza Chacón, Francisco Díaz, Juan Fragoso, and Bartolomé Hidalgo de Agüero), they collectively published sixteen separate treatises, most of which were republished numerous times through the following century. Juan Calvo's *Primera y segunda parte de la cirugía universal*, for example, first published in

Castilian (in Seville) in 1580, underwent at least ten re-editions in Castilian, as well as two in French, and was still reprinted as late as 1703.[19] Juan Fragoso's similar surgical compendium (also entitled *Cirugía universal*), first published in 1581, was still being republished as late as 1713.

Learned surgeons could be found working and publishing texts all across Spain. Rather than discuss each individual in sequence, I have chosen to focus on them as a group and to analyze their work thematically. Brief individual biographies may be found in the appendix. The first chapter examines the particular Spanish context in which these men worked, giving the background not only of medieval education and licensing but more specifically of the Spanish practices for training and licensing. Beginning with education, it examines the rise of universities and the emergent medieval separation of physicians from other kinds of practitioners. This division was slowly narrowed by medieval surgeons who sought to create their own learned and text-based profession. Surgery later became taught in universities as well, which encouraged the bifurcation between the learned surgeons (university educated and Latinate) and apprentice-trained surgeons (literate but not Latinate, called *romancista* in Spanish). It then turns to the complex issues of licensure and the rise of the médico y cirujano as a distinct type of surgeon.

Chapter 2 focuses on the set of learned surgeons whose work and careers form the core of the book. It examines their professional and personal biographies, narrated within the ties or networks that connected them. It argues that while these men formed a series of loose networks, they retained distinct differences between them. Learned surgeons were a very small elite of practitioners, who did not all follow the same path. They were from a variety of backgrounds, gained their experience in varying ways, and followed their own career paths and personal interests. In addition, this chapter examines connections between surgeons and other intellectuals, including print references to each other's work and the important intellectual networks centered in Seville and Valencia.

The third chapter examines the texts written by these learned surgeons, which were largely in the vernacular. Here again, there is a complex context both to the history of surgical (vernacular) texts vis-à-vis medical (Latin) texts and to the history of printing in Spain. This chapter also puts these sixteenth-century texts into context with their medieval forerunners, demonstrating the continuities as well as innovations within their structure and approach.

The final two chapters examine the innovations and refinements of knowledge and practice found in the work of these surgeons. Chapter 4 focuses on two case studies of how empiricism was used to refine knowledge and treatment. The first case study examines in detail the famous debate, carried out in print, between Bartolomé Hidalgo de Agüero and Juan Fragoso over wound treatment (wet vs. dry healing). It explains the context of the dispute as well as the influence of their ideas through the next century and beyond. The second case study looks at neurosurgery, specifically the practice of trepanation. Here experience and experiment were paramount in improving trepans (the tools) and the understanding of how and when to use them successfully.

The final chapter turns from refinement or improvement of knowledge and practice to the ways surgeons developed entirely new expertise. This included two categories: bodily ailments new to surgeons and bodily ailments that newly emerged in the sixteenth century. In the former category were things that had not previously been codified as part of the surgeon's expertise, such as urology and legal medicine, which included both forensic (cause of death) and other legal questions that called upon medical expertise, such as fertility and paternity. In the second category was the development of both theory and practice for entirely new problems such as gunshot wounds and new diseases, including typhus and *morbo gálico* (the French disease or Great Pox).[20] In response to all these disorders of the body, learned surgeons developed and applied theory, practiced new techniques, and sought to pass on their knowledge to later generations by compiling and publishing texts.

Notes

1 Roy Porter and Mikuláš Teich, eds., *The Renaissance in National Context* (New York: Cambridge University Press, 1992), 1.

2 Two recent works examining changes in medicine in German lands are Hannah Murphy, *A New Order of Medicine: The Rise of Physicians in Reformation Nuremberg* (Pittsburgh: University of Pittsburgh Press, 2019); Erik A. Heinrichs, *Plague, Print, and the Reformation: The German Reform of Healing, 1473–1573* (New York: Routledge, 2018); For other changes in medicine in this era, see Gianna Pomata, "Observation Rising: Birth of an Epistemic Genre, 1500–1650," in *Histories of Scientific Observation*, ed. Lorraine Daston and Elizabeth Lunbeck (Chicago, IL: University of Chicago Press, 2011), 45–80; Paolo Savoia, *Gaspare Tagliacozzi and Early Modern Surgery: Faces, Men, and Pain* (New York: Routledge, 2019).

3 Domenico Bertoloni Meli and Cynthia Klestinec, "Renaissance Surgery Between Learning and Craft," *Journal of the History of Medicine and Allied Sciences* 72, no. 1 (2017): 1, https://doi.org/10.1093/jhmas/jrw043. See also the articles in this journal special edition. Other recent work on surgery includes Savoia, *Gaspare Tagliacozzi and Early Modern Surgery*; Cynthia Klestinec, "Vesalius among the Surgeons," *Journal of Medieval and Early Modern Studies* 48, no. 1 (January 1, 2018): 125–51, https://doi.org/10.1215/10829636-4280882; Elaine Leong, "Learning Medicine by the Book: Reading and Writing Surgical Manuals in Early Modern London," *BJHS Themes* 5 (2020): 93–110, https://doi.org/10.1017/bjt.2020.7; Hannah Murphy, "Skin and Disease in Early Modern Medicine: Jan Jessen's *De Cute, et Cutaneis Affectibus* (1601)," *Bulletin of the History of Medicine* 94, no. 2 (2020): 179–214, https://doi.org/10.1353/bhm.2020.0034; Donatella Bartolini, "On the Borders: Surgeons and Their Activities in the Venetian State (1540–1640)," *Medical History* 59, no. 01 (2015): 83–100, https://doi.org/10.1017/mdh.2014.72.

4 Marie-Christine Pouchelle, *The Body and Surgery in the Middle Ages* (New Brunswick, NJ: Rutgers University Press, 1990), 13; Nancy G Siraisi, *Taddeo Alderotti and His Pupils: Two Generations of Italian Medical Learning* (Princeton, NJ: Princeton University Press, 2019), 56–7, https://doi.org/10.1515/9780691198163.

5 Murphy, "Skin and Disease in Early Modern Medicine," 179.

6 Jerome J. Bylebyl, "The School of Padua: Humanistic Medicine in the Sixteenth Century," in *Health, Medicine and Mortality in the Sixteenth Century*, ed. Charles Webster (New York: Cambridge University Press, 1979), 354.

7 Christelle Rabier, "Medicalizing the Surgical Trade, 1650–1820: Workers, Knowledge, Markets and Politics," in *The Palgrave Handbook of the History of Surgery*, ed. Thomas Schlich (London: Palgrave Macmillan, 2018), 74.

8 Bjørn Okholm Skaarup, *Anatomy and Anatomists in Early Modern Spain* (Burlington, VT: Ashgate, 2015), 119.
9 There is no bibliography specifically compiling vernacular surgical (or medical) texts across Europe, though Solomon includes an excellent bibliography for Spain. Michael Solomon, *Fictions of Well-Being: Sickly Readers and Vernacular Medical Writing in Late Medieval and Early Modern Spain* (Philadelphia: University of Pennsylvania Press, 2010).
10 Lucinda McCray Beier, "Seventeenth-Century English Surgery: The Casebook of Joseph Binns," in *Medical Theory, Surgical Practice* (New York: Routledge, 1992), 48–84; Lauren Kassell, "Casebooks in Early Modern England: Medicine, Astrology, and Written Records," *Bulletin of the History of Medicine* 88, no. 4 (2014): 595–625.
11 Gianna Pomata, "Sharing Cases: The *Observationes* in Early Modern Medicine," *Early Science and Medicine* 15, no. 3 (2010): 193–236, https://doi.org/10.1163/157338210X493932.
12 There are a handful of texts in English that discuss some or all of these men, while the vast Spanish language scholarship is evident in the bibliography. An early seminal work was Luis S. Granjel, *Cirugía Española Del Renacimiento* (Salamanca: Universidad de Salamanca, 1968); English language studies include Kristy Wilson Bowers, "Tradition and Innovation in Spanish Medicine: Bartolomé Hidalgo de Agüero and the Vía Particular," *Sixteenth Century Journal* XLI, no. I (2010): 29–47; Charles Donald O'Malley, "Dionisio Daza Chacon," in *Medizingeschichte in Unserer Zeit. Festgabe Fur Edith Heischkel-Artelt Und Walter Artelt Zum 65. Geburtstag.*, ed. Hans-Heinz Eulner et al. (Stuttgart: Ferndinand Enke Verlag, 1971), 160–70; Michele L. Clouse, *Medicine, Government and Public Health in Philip II's Spain: Shared Interests, Competing Authorities* (Burlington, VT: Ashgate, 2011); Skaarup, *Anatomy and Anatomists in Early Modern Spain.*
13 John Edwards, *The Spain of the Catholic Monarchs, 1474–1520* (Malden, MA: Blackwell Publishers, 2000), 261–65.
14 Edwards, 261.
15 Edwards, 266–67; Martin Biersack, "The Adoption of Humanism in Catholic Spain (1470–1520)," *Reformation & Renaissance Review* 21, no. 1 (January 2, 2019): 27–8.
16 Thomas James Dandelet, *Spanish Rome, 1500–1700* (New Haven, CT: Yale University Press, 2008); Miles Pattenden and Piers Baker-Bates (eds.), *The Spanish Presence in Sixteenth-Century Italy: Images of Iberia* (Burlington, VT: Ashgate Publishing, 2015); Michael Jacob Levin, *Agents of Empire: Spanish Ambassadors in Sixteenth-Century Italy* (Ithaca, NY: Cornell University Press, 2005).
17 José Luis Fresquet Febrer, "La práctica médica en los textos quirúrgicos españoles en el siglo XVIII," *Dynamis: Acta Hispanica Ad Medicinae Scientiarumque Historiam Illustrandam* 22 (2002): 251–77; Jose Luis Fresquet Febrer, ed., *Juan Calvo y la Cirugía Valenciana del Siglo XVI: Simposio 2002 Sobre la Historia de la Medicina* (València: Editorial Denes, 2002); Pedro Conde Parrado, "«Por el orden de Celso»: aspectos de la influencia del 'De medicina' en la cirugía europea del Renacimiento," *Dynamis: Acta Hispanica ad Medicinae Scientiarumque Historiam Illustrandam* 28 (2008): 217–242; Joaquín Herrera Dávila, *El Hospital del Cardenal de Sevilla y el Doctor Hidalgo de Agüero* (Sevilla: Fundación de Cultura Andaluza, 2010); María Luz López Terrada, "Médicos, Cirujanos, Boticarios y Albéitares," in *Historia de La Ciencia y de La Técnica En La Corona de Castilla*, ed. Luis García Ballester, vol. III (Valladolid: Junta de Castilla y León, Consejería de Educación y Cultura, 2002), 161–85.
18 See, for example, the discussions in José L. Fresquet Febrer, "El Interés del Estudio de la Cirugía en la Monarquía Hispánica (s. XVI)," in *Más allá de la Leyenda Negra: España y la Revolución Científica = Beyond the Black Legend: Spain and the Scientific Revolution*, ed. Víctor Navarro Brotons and William Eamon (València: Universidad de València, Inst. de Historia de la Ciencia y Documentación López Piñero, 2007), 295–306; Fresquet Febrer, "La práctica médica en los textos quirúrgicos españoles en el siglo XVIII"; Alfredo Moreno-Egea, "Aportaciones de los cirujanos españoles del Renacimiento," *Revista Hispanoamericana de Hernia* 4, no. 4 (October 2016): 163–72, https://doi.org/10.1016/j.rehah.2016.04.001; Granjel, *Cirugía Española Del Renacimiento*, 24–7; Luis S. Granjel, *La*

Medicina Española Renacentista, Historia General de La Medicina Española, II (Salamanca: Universidad de Salamanca, 1980), 213–29; José María López Piñero, *Ciencia y técnica en la sociedad española de los siglos XVI y XVII* (Barcelona: Labor Universitaria, 1979), 360–68. The latter three larger studies do mention a number of other surgeons but focus primarily on the works of these particular men. A brief discussion in English is provided by Fielding H. Garrison, "An Epitome of the History of Spanish Medicine," *Bulletin of the New York Academy of Medicine* 7, no. 8 (1931): 604–5.

19 José López Piñero et al., *Diccionario Histórico de La Ciencia Moderna En España*, 1a ed., vol. I (A–L) (Barcelona: Península, 1983), 160–1.

20 These terms were used to refer to a disease that became widespread in the late fifteenth century and was known by many different names. It is today most often equated with syphilis, but not all historians agree with this as a retrospective diagnosis. I therefore use the Spanish term most commonly found in the sixteenth century, which was morbo gálico.

1

PHYSICIANS AND SURGEONS

Medical Learning and Licensing

Juan Fragoso began his publishing career in 1566 with a Latin book on medical simples, *Catalogus simplicium medicamentorum*. Four years later he published his first work on surgery, *Erotemas chirurgicos*, which he expanded and revised over the next decade into a larger compendium, *Cirugía universal*. This latter text included treatises on a variety of topics, including anatomy, pharmacy, and legal medicine (which included legal issues such as determining cause of death, fertility, impotency, and the legitimacy of offspring). These were all modern topics for sixteenth-century surgeons, reflecting an inquisitive mind and an individual who kept abreast of current events and the work of colleagues from across Europe. But Fragoso's work was also steeped in the traditions of classical medicine. The last treatise added to the *Cirugía universal* was a compilation of Hippocratic aphorisms related to surgery. He offered each of these in Latin with Castilian translation and a brief explanation. In a further nod to tradition, Fragoso turned to Galen for these explanations, citing books and chapters from the illustrious Roman throughout the treatise. In fact, Fragoso provided copious citations through all his works, reflecting the ancient, medieval, and contemporary authors to whom he was indebted. In the prefatory material of the original *Erotemas* is a list of fifty-seven authorities referred to in the text, ranging from Hippocrates to renowned Spanish royal physician Francisco Valles (known as "the divine" for his erudition), from Aristotle to Vesalius. Fragoso, like all learned surgeons, was well aware of the historical traditions he had inherited as well as the contemporary intellectual shifts he was contributing to.

Ancient and Medieval Surgery

Surgery was always an integral part of medicine and yet also always a distinct set of knowledge and skills. While historians have long emphasized the latter, particularly in the form of a premodern professional divide between physicians and surgeons,

DOI: 10.4324/9781003291060-2

the ancient texts that were foundational to premodern medicine make no such professional distinctions. The Hippocratic corpus includes such texts as *De fracturis* (On Fractures) and *De capitus vulneribus* (On Head Wounds), which offer insight into treatment of specific physical conditions, but do not distinguish those who undertake them as distinct practitioners.[1] The renunciation of cutting (for stone) in the Hippocratic Oath has been interpreted in various ways: most broadly as setting surgery apart from physic, but most narrowly as merely advising against deliberate creation of wounds as a part of healing.[2] Celsus, the second-century Roman author (though not practitioner), defines medicine as "divided into three parts: one being that which cures through diet, another through medicaments, and the third by hand," apparently laying out the fields of physic, pharmacy, and surgery, but he likewise does not suggest these should be utilized by separate practitioners.[3] Nonetheless, historians have credited Celsus with establishing "surgery as a coherent category of medical thinking," and even as both physic and surgery may have been practiced by the same person, the knowledge and skills required for each continued to be treated separately in texts.[4]

The textual tradition is all that remains to us from this ancient era, as well as many of the ensuing centuries. We can trace surviving texts (and fragments) much more than individual practitioners. These ancient texts were absorbed and expanded upon by medical writers in the Islamic world, returning to European scholars with the translation movement that flourished from the twelfth century on in both Iberia and southern Italy. Medical texts were at the forefront of these translations, as generations of medical scholars in the Islamic world had absorbed ancient Greek and Latin texts, expanding and refining them according to their own experiences. Among the influential Islamic authors were several who included treatises on surgery within or alongside their works on physic, including Ibn Sina (Avicenna, 980–1037), al-Rāzī (Rhazes, c. 865–925), and al-Zāhrāwi (Albucasis, c. 936–1013). While the extent to which these men actually (or routinely) undertook some of the surgical practices they wrote about is unclear, their texts were nonetheless highly influential.[5] Translation and use of some of this Islamic work are earliest evident at Salerno (Italy), seen in the work of Constantine the African and the compilation known as the Trotula.[6] These textual traditions were then also codified by medieval teaching masters into standardized curricula. Early medical licensing regulations, which rulers began to implement in the same era, likewise pointed to knowledge as paramount over skills.[7] Though medical learning and licensing came to be entwined in the Middle Ages, here we will focus on just learning and the textual tradition for surgery, turning to consider licensing separately.

Medieval Education

The earliest European universities, including Bologna (1088), Paris (1150), and Oxford (1167), led the way for the rapid expansion in such foundations in the thirteenth. In Castile, early *studia generalia* included Palencia (1208), Salamanca (1218), Valladolid (1241), and Sevilla (1254); in the Crown of Aragon, foundations included Montpellier (1289, though the territory and university were no longer part of Aragon after 1344), Lérida (Lleida, 1300), and Perpignan (1350). To round out the peninsula, Coimbra (Portugal) established a university in 1290, and in Muslim Granada, the Emir Yusuf I established a Madrasah or mosque school in 1349 where similar topics of philosophy, law, medicine, and theology were studied.[8]

Medical studies were not the driving purpose of any medieval universities but came to be included in most. Records of instruction and attendance at medical courses in these early centuries are often irregular, however, and do not give us a full picture of what was taught and to how many. García Ballester has pointed out, for example, that while the University of Salamanca's royal privilege (1254) called for "two masters of physic," there is no clear evidence of actual medical teaching until the mid-fourteenth century.[9] In Lérida, McVaugh has found that the first medical teaching master was often called away from the university to attend to the royal family, and the *studium* itself was shut for a number of years between 1304 and 1310 due to a dispute over the appointment of its masters.[10] Despite the sporadic and inconclusive nature of these early records, it is nonetheless clear that as medical faculties became established in universities, the emergence of educated physicians from them increased the demand for such learned practitioners.[11]

The development of a distinct textual tradition for surgery also arose in the thirteenth century. Educated and skilled Italian surgeons, including Teodorico Borgognoni (1205–96/8), Bruno Longobucco (c.1200–c.1286), and Guglielmo da Saliceto (1210–77), produced Latin texts devoted exclusively to surgery, creating a body of knowledge still entwined with but distinct from physic.[12] Lanfranc of Milan (c.1250–1306), a student of Guglielmo da Saliceto, moved to Paris in the late thirteenth century where he taught surgery and wrote his own text, *Chirurgia magna* (1296). Michael McVaugh who has closely studied this early textual tradition refers to this as the rise of rational surgery, a growing movement of using written texts to both consolidate knowledge and to lift the intellectual status of surgery as resting on both theory and practice. By the fourteenth century, surgical teaching was offered sporadically at Paris and Montpellier and more regularly at Bologna, Padua, Ferrara, Pavia, and Turin in Italy. In Aragon, the *studium* of Lérida offered surgical courses from 1300, while in Valencia an *Estudi de Cirugía* offered similar surgical study where no university yet existed.[13]

Educated surgeons in the fourteenth century continued to teach and defend surgery as a learned endeavor, based in ancient theory but expanded by experience. Henri de Mondeville (1260–1320), who taught anatomy and surgery at Montpellier before moving to Paris as royal surgeon and teaching master, is one of the earliest for whom we can trace his medical education (Montpellier and Paris) and surgical studies (Bologna).[14] Though Mondeville died before finishing his great surgical text, his contemporary Guy de Chauliac (c.1300–68) produced a more definitive and influential text. That they wrote in Latin signaled both their erudition and the existence of an audience for such learned works. These physician-surgeons became models in many ways for the later learned surgeons of the sixteenth century. In fact, Chauliac was still considered foundational enough for Juan Calvo to produce a new Castilian edition of his *Chirurgia* as late as 1596, long after he had published several editions of his own surgical text, one that was arguably meant to replace Chauliac's.

Any discussion of surgical teaching in late medieval universities must broaden to acknowledge anatomical studies, which also came into universities in the fourteenth century, based in part on the new text of Mondino de Luzzi, *Anathomia corporis humani* (1316). The connections between anatomy and surgery seem obvious to modern scholars, but in this earlier era, they were much more tenuous. The impetus for anatomical studies was more directly tied to postmortem pathology and humoral theory than to surgical practice.[15] While anatomical lecturers (and authors) often practiced surgery, the incorporation of anatomical chairs in universities did not necessarily bring surgical chairs as well. Instead, in some places, by the turn of the sixteenth century, anatomical teaching became tied to botanical teaching as universities created chairs of anatomy and simples, responsible for anatomical dissection in colder winter months and botanical fieldwork in warmer ones.[16] Even Andreas Vesalius, arguably the most influential anatomist of the sixteenth century, was neither trained nor skilled as a surgeon, though his initial position at Padua was a lectureship in surgery, and his later imperial appointment put him on the battlefield, treating wounded soldiers in the Habsburg-Valois Wars.[17] Nonetheless, anatomy and surgery remained connected in their focus on the physical body, both sound and unsound. Learned surgical treatises of the sixteenth century, particularly after Vesalius's influential publication, increasingly included discussion of anatomy. In addition, the continued production of learned anatomical texts helped reinforce the importance of Galenic theory for knowing the best approaches to heal the wounds, fractures, and abscesses that surgeons were called to treat.

Medical Humanism

The fifteenth century gave rise to humanism, the intellectual movement that sought a return to ancient written sources, analyzed with fresh eyes (so to speak) through new forms of textual study, linguistics, and philology. The humanist program reached medical studies by the late fifteenth century, prompting some, such as Niccolò Leoniceno, to see the "Arabized" medical texts of Avicenna and others as unacceptably filtering or altering the original ancient knowledge. The "destructive criticism" of humanists, rejecting medieval as well as Arabic translations soon was complemented by literature denouncing the errors of ancients as well.[18] The spread of the printing press from the mid-fifteenth century on enabled the circulation of these critiques, as well as new "cleaner" editions of ancient writers to circulate. Scholars began publishing new editions not only of Hippocrates and Galen but also of other previously neglected ancients such as Celsus and Paul of Aegina.[19] In the early sixteenth century, scholars in France and Italy refused to teach with the older Arabized texts, turning instead to new Latin translations of Graeco-Roman learning. Medical writing expanded and diversified as a result, though the influence of Islamic scholars did not diminish.[20]

As humanism entered universities, it challenged and eventually replaced the older scholastic tradition. In Spain, the universities most associated with humanism were those in Valencia and Alcalá de Henares (where the first polyglot Bible was produced in the early decades of the sixteenth century), though humanism penetrated into at least parts of all universities by the sixteenth century. Salamanca provides an interesting case of embracing humanism without rejecting translated medical texts. Although it was the academic home of Antonio de Nebrija, the great Castilian humanist and linguist whose publications on Latin and Castilian grammar were unsurpassed in influence, the medical school remained "Arabized" in orientation, teaching Galenic medicine through Arabic writers, most especially Avicenna.[21] Similarly, sixteenth-century learned surgeons embraced the work of medical humanists alongside, rather than in place of, Islamic and medieval texts. They were clearly familiar with and cited a wide range of humanist scholars such as Niccolò Leoniceno, Giovanni Manardo, and Antonio Musa Brassavola, along with continuing to quote from Avicenna and Albucasis. Ancient authors whose work was newly recovered, such as Celsus and Paul of Aegina, were likewise favored alongside Galen and Hippocrates.[22]

The inclusion of such a wide range of previous scholarship in the texts of learned surgeons may reflect two purposes—to show their intellectual legitimacy and to pass on as much knowledge as possible to their audience. For despite the seemingly promising development of surgery as a learned profession embedded in university training in the thirteenth and fourteenth centuries, by the early sixteenth century, that promise was only partially fulfilled. Surgery was taught in some universities but remained separate from physic. Within universities, surgical courses of study were held inferior in status to courses in internal medicine and did not typically draw many students.[23] Examining Berengario da Carpi's success and prominence teaching surgery at Bologna, Roger French argues that he was an exception and that "surgical teaching was not highly regarded, not popular with the Italian students and perhaps only tolerated at the academic level of the *studium* because it brought foreign students into the town."[24] Surgeons with university degrees, then, remained a relatively small elite group, which in turn makes the significant number of Spanish learned surgeons all more noteworthy.

Equally important to the continued growth and advancement of the professional surgeon were the hospitals where many trained and then practiced. While the full medicalization of hospitals and their association as teaching centers for professional surgery is often tied to the Enlightenment, medical hospitals as sites of teaching existed from the late Middle Ages.[25] Among the most famous teaching hospitals in Castile were those of the Monastery of Santa María of Guadalupe, founded in the thirteenth century. The early records of an attached hospital date to 1329, and by the fifteenth century, the monastery housed three hospitals, one each for males, females, and religious.[26] As these foundations grew in repute, they attracted both well-known practitioners to serve there and younger scholars seeking further experience and training.[27] Well-known practitioners who learned and worked there include Francisco Arceo (one of the learned surgeons studied here); Francisco Hernández, who was later appointed as royal *Protomédico* for Philip II and sent to New Spain to license practitioners and survey the flora and fauna there; and Benito Bustamante de Paz, who studied in both Spain and Italy and later wrote a well-known Latin commentary on Hippocrates.[28]

In sixteenth-century Spain, hospitals retained an amalgam of charitable and medical services. Small, specialized hospitals proliferated in cities and towns, many of them with only a handful of beds and dedicated to particular populations (women, priests, confraternity members) or sufferers from particular diseases (leprosy and morbo gálico each had their own institutions; plague hospitals were often buildings temporarily repurposed during an outbreak).[29] Over the course of the century, royal foundations increased, but overall numbers of hospitals decreased in Castile as the monarchs (both Charles V and Philip II) embraced hospital consolidation. Such efforts began the century before in Aragon, as Fernando I oversaw hospital reductions in cities including Barcelona, Zaragoza, and Valencia.[30] Consolidation was generally motivated by efforts to better regulate poor relief and the financial stability of institutions but had the additional effect of expanding the scope of medical care in hospitals.[31] Cities in both Aragon and Castile continued to host multiple hospitals that offered medical care, usually including a General Hospital where patients could seek care for a variety of problems and surgeons often gained training. Specialized hospitals also remained to treat women, the mentally disabled, and the previously mentioned diseases.

Surgeons first trained and then often worked in hospitals. All of the learned surgeons discussed here had some connection to hospital practice, though Bartolomé Hidalgo de Agüero was the only one whose entire career was spent at one, the Hospital del Cardinal in Seville. To offer an assortment of other examples, Juan Calvo, best known as a teacher of surgery in Valencia, recounts a story of his experience with a rarely used type of cautery. Having once previously seen the surgeon Jerónimo Murillo use it successfully in the hospital in Zaragoza, presumably while he was in training, Calvo many years later was able to successfully use it on a patient he was then treating at the General Hospital of Valencia.[32] His framing of this personal anecdote points to both the delicate nature of some treatments (requiring clear knowledge of when and how to apply them) and the importance of hospital settings for some types of treatment. Dionisio Daza Chacón, who held a variety of positions affiliated with the royal family, spent six years as head surgeon at the Royal Hospital in Valladolid. At the death of the previous surgeon there, Princess Juana, acting as regent at the time, appointed Daza Chacón to the post. Hospital administrators, whether concerned with ensuring the best candidate was chosen or simply to assert their power against the crown, demanded an open competition for the prestigious position. Daza Chacón won the position against fourteen rivals, among them another learned surgeon under consideration here, Francisco Díaz.[33] Díaz, after not getting this hospital job, moved to Burgos and was a municipal surgeon there for seven years before moving to Madrid to seek a court position. Presumably, his time in Burgos included work in a city hospital, for he offers a negative view of them. In his *Compendio de Cirugía* (1575) written in the form of a dialogue between doctor and student, Díaz has the experienced doctor denounce his dissatisfaction with hospital work as difficult because there are too many patients and so few resources that one cannot spend the time and effort on each patient that one should.[34]

Regulating Medicine

The regulation or licensing of medical practitioners developed in the same era as the universities, from the twelfth century on. Here again, the early records remain sporadic, with King Roger of Sicily acknowledged as the first to promulgate royal regulations in 1140.[35] The growth of universities created an important path to professional legitimacy, but this increasingly overlapped (and conflicted) with licensing regulations enacted by both royal and municipal authorities. Where guild systems became entrenched, these too provided assurances of members' fitness for practice.[36] Medical regulation across Europe seems to have remained largely local and often disputed between various corporations: guilds, colleges, university masters, practicing physicians, and civic leaders.

Given the limited embrace of surgery by universities, professional associations of surgeons, in the form of guilds or colleges, played an important role in distinguishing and protecting the status of learned surgeons as above barbers or barber-surgeons and on par with physicians. The London Fellowship of Surgeons, established in mid-fourteenth century, folded the earliest, joining the Company of Barbers in 1540, while the thirteenth century Parisian College of Saint-Côme for master surgeons successfully held its own against the city's physicians until the eighteenth. The Valencian *Colegio de Barberos y Cirujanos*, established in 1433, retained learned status as it was absorbed by the University of Valencia after its founding in 1499. A more unusual case was the *Colegio de Médicos y Cirujanos* of Zaragoza, which had been originally established by surgeons and barbers in the city (as the *Cofradía de San Cosme y San Damián y San Valentín*) who agreed to serve at the *Hospital de Nuestra Señora de Gracia*. Within a decade, physicians began joining the college, which later maintained control over all medical practitioners in the city, independent even of royal efforts to control regulation by establishing a *Protomédico* in 1592.[37]

Though licensing exams initially did not emphasize or require university training, over time such learning was increasingly required for physicians. Only in some regions, notably Aragon, was university training enforced for surgeons, who were more often examined for skill. In France, for example, early fourteenth-century royal regulations of King Philip IV stipulated surgery as a craft, with no theoretical or textual study required.[38] This regulation contravened the work of the royal surgeon Henri de Mondeville, to whom McVaugh attributes an early effort "to convince the academic physicians of Paris that it would do their discipline no harm to introduce *operatio manualis* into medical training, and…to convince empiric surgeons that their practice could only be truly successful if they first obtained a theoretical grounding in anatomy, physiology, and pathology."[39] Mondeville was not successful in getting support from King Philip IV for these ideas. Two centuries later, however, a different King Philip, Philip II of Spain, took up this same cause, expanding surgical studies within universities and for all medical students.

In supporting academic surgery, Philip II was building on medieval foundations in the Crown of Aragon. To understand this context, it is necessary to again go back to the thirteenth century, before the Crowns of Castile and Aragon were united.

Those territorial differences, marked by differing legislative bodies (*cortes*, *corts*) and laws (*fueros*, *furs*) remained entrenched through the sixteenth century and beyond. Aragon was at the forefront of regulating medical and surgical education. The early regulations, promulgated by King Alfons III (1285–91) in 1289, delegated licensing control to city officials. Control slowly shifted in some places, Valencia for example, to physicians themselves as they increasingly made up the licensing boards in cities. By 1329, Alfons IV (1327–36), working with the *corts* of Valencia, refined regulations there to include a requirement for university study for all practitioners, surgeons, and physicians. This was extended throughout the remainder of Aragon by 1359.[40] Similarly, as noted earlier, in Zaragoza physicians joined the confraternity of surgeons and barbers, and the renamed Colegio de Médicos y Cirujanos then gained control of regulating medical practitioners there. Thus, we see the emergence of an interconnected regulatory system with varying input from crown, municipalities, physicians, and universities. The same multiplicity of voices was found in Castile, though it should be noted that in both regions, this multiplicity led more often to conflict than to cooperation.[41]

In Castile, regulation of physicians and surgeons had also been granted to local *alcaldes* (town mayors) in the thirteenth century by Fernando III (1201–52) and Alphonso X (1252–84).[42] In the fifteenth century, rulers began to assert more direct control over medicine, culminating in the creation of a permanent regulatory institution, the *Tribunal del Protomedicato* under Isabel and Fernando in 1477.[43] The Protomedicato held power for examining and licensing various medical professions, including physicians, surgeons, apothecaries, spicers, bonesetters, and others engaged in related health professions.[44] This insertion of royal prerogative into medicine was not uncontested, and conflict between the crown and cities continued throughout the sixteenth century.[45] Despite these challenges, the Protomedicato continued to function with waxing and waning powers, until its eventual suppression in 1822.

Over the course of the sixteenth century, under both Charles V (r. 1516–56) and Philip II (r. 1556–98), the Protomedicato underwent a number of changes, both large and small, as a result of both new ideas in medicine and of the constant negotiation between city leaders, university leaders, and the crown.[46] Significant changes during the reign of Charles V both limited and expanded the Protomedicato. In response to petitions from the municipal representatives in the Cortes, Charles agreed to limit the professions it regulated to just physicians, surgeons, apothecaries, and barbers, leaving out spice dealers, herbalists, bonesetters, midwives, and other practitioners who now became relegated to the broader medical marketplace and more directly under the control of local officials. In addition, he agreed to limit the geographic reach of the board to an area of five leagues around court. This likewise seems to have been in response to complaints from the Cortes and petitions from municipal authorities to have more local regulatory oversight themselves.[47]

While this did leave cities more room to regulate local medical professionals, it did not entirely circumscribe the geographic reach of royal licensing, as the court was mobile and moved periodically between various royal residences. In addition, many practitioners willingly traveled to the court from great distances in order to be licensed, gaining thereby royal approval to practice anywhere in the realm.[48] Alongside these technical contractions of oversight, however, Charles V also oversaw the expansion of the Protomedicato outside Castile, establishing additional Protomedicatos in the Aragonese territories of Valencia, Navarre, Catalonia, Mallorca, and Naples.[49] This expansion was met with even greater resistance, as a rejection of outside influence. Thus, in several of these areas, the power of the Protomédico was in name only, as entrenched guild and municipal interests continued to push back against the encroach of royal power.

Regulating Education in Spain

Charles V's reign also saw changes in surgical education, both what was available and what was required. The incorporation of both surgery and anatomy in Spanish universities, as noted earlier, was led by Aragonese universities of Lérida and Valencia. Lérida began teaching surgery in the early fourteenth century, while Valencia did so from its establishment in 1499. At that time, Valencia's long-standing school of surgery, the *Estudi de Cirugia*, was incorporated into the university along with a chair of medicine and another chair of anatomy and simples (materia medica).[50] The Estudi had already been teaching anatomy, having received royal privilege to dissect cadavers in 1477, but the chair of anatomy and simples at the new university was filled by anatomists deeply influenced by the ideas of Vesalius, including Luis Collado and Pedro Jimeno. [51] The University of Valencia subsequently trained the men who became chairs of anatomy at Castilian universities, including Cosme de Medina at Salamanca and Pedro Jimeno at Alcalá de Henares.[52] Castilian universities slowly added chairs in anatomy and/or surgery throughout the sixteenth century. The initial push came from Charles V, who first began requiring both expanded coursework and expanded supervised practical training for medical degrees in the 1530s.[53] By 1551, Charles mandated the teaching of anatomy in Castilian universities in addition to supporting dissections by authorizing universities to procure bodies of executed criminals for study.[54] Both Valladolid and Alcalá were already offering anatomical instruction before that date but gained permanent chairs then. Surgery tended to lag behind anatomy in the universities, though here again, some professors of medicine taught aspects of surgery in their courses. The creation of surgical chairs in universities came under mandates from Philip II.

Over the second half of the century, Philip II continued the practices set out by his father of royal intervention in both medical licensing and education. Over the course of his reign, he slowly but successfully amended the composition and duties of the *Protomedicato*, extending its power and reach to new areas. For example, despite establishing Madrid as a permanent court in 1561, Philip still traveled frequently, visiting various parts of his domains. He continued to bring medical personnel with him, empowering them with uncovering and punishing false licenses or unlicensed practitioners in these locales. He further expanded the offices of the Protomedicato to the New World, to Portugal after he became ruler there in 1580, and to the Kingdom of Aragon in 1592. Within Castile, Philip issued several mandates over the course of his reign in an ongoing effort to better regulate medical practice. As pointed out by María Luz López Terrada, this was necessary not simply as a means for Philip (or, for that matter, for local municipal leaders) to expand their power and interests but was also a response to a continually expanding medical marketplace clearly in need of regulation.[55]

Philip II is often remembered for another set of regulations, the restrictions aimed at preventing Protestant ideas from circulating in his realms. These came in the form of regulations on printing, the creation of a Spanish Index of Forbidden Books, and restrictions on foreign study. While the innovative ideas of foreign humanists, such as Erasmus and Ficino, were popular and circulated widely in the first part of the sixteenth century, by mid-century, the perceived threat posed by reformed religious ideas prompted Philip II to issue this series of royal mandates aimed at preventing their further spread.[56] The Council of Castile gained control over licenses for printing as well as oversight on the importation of foreign works. Students from Castile studying abroad were ordered to return home within months, and study at foreign universities was forbidden, with the exception of Rome, Bologna, Naples, and Coimbra.[57] On the surface, this restrictive legislation, coupled with an active Inquisition working to root out Protestantism within Castile, has been interpreted as closing down Spain intellectually, preventing scholars from participating in the broader intellectual movements. In the past, historians of science pointed to these efforts as preventing Spanish participation in the scientific revolution, an interpretation soundly dismissed in more recent scholarship.[58] The restrictions (both on publications and on studying abroad) pertained only to the Kingdom of Castile, not to the Crown of Aragon, which encompassed a significant expanse of territory. These territories (Aragon, Catalonia, Valencia, Navarre), many of them sitting along the Mediterranean seaboard, held deep and long-standing political, economic, and cultural ties across the Mediterranean. These ties created the entanglements between the peninsulas of Spain and Italy, enabling Rome, Bologna, and Naples to be perceived as safely Catholic. To enact (and enforce) similar legislation in any of the territories of Aragon, Philip II would have had to personally visit and gain the support of the legislative bodies of each, which he did not attempt. Thus, the peninsula was never intellectually closed, not in any meaningful way. The continued circulation of people, and especially texts and ideas between Spain and the rest of Europe, particularly for science and medicine, has been well documented.[59] While these censorship efforts were perhaps successful in preventing a religious reformation in Spain, the intellectual culture, particularly the elite culture of universities, continued to hold a wide continuum of views from conservatives holding fast to the old ideas to innovators pushing for the new.[60]

At roughly the same time that he worked to restrict access to foreign universities for study, Philip II also began intervening in university curricula at home. In response to a petition from city leaders in 1566, he ordered the University of Salamanca to add a chair of surgery.[61] The first to hold this chair was one of the learned surgeons under consideration here, Andrés Alcázar. Philip II later mandated similar inclusions at the Universities of Valladolid and Alcalá de Henares.[62] In doing so, he required that all medical students, whether intending to practice surgery or not, had to complete classes in surgery. These decrees initiated a series of changes in requirements for medical students, culminating in the 1593 pragmatic, which reorganized the Protomedicato and, in particular, decreed that no candidate for a surgical license could be examined who did not have a full bachelor of arts degree, three medical courses, and two years of practical training alongside a licensed surgeon.[63] This effectively tightened the requirements for a royal license, as it amended earlier legislation that did not require surgical candidates to have a full degree but had merely required their attendance in medical as well as surgical lectures.[64]

According to crown policies, then, we find throughout the sixteenth century increased regulations on education and licensing that pushed surgery into becoming a more learned field, one studied by anyone wishing to study medicine at all. This would appear a fairly dramatic change, one that would effectively eliminate (over time) most of the traditional (apprentice-trained) surgeons. Supporting this movement was the generation of médico y cirujanos, who are the focus of this study and who were already practicing by the time Philip began issuing mandates. They were the leading edge of a movement to lift the training and status of surgeons, whose vernacular texts were meant to act as a bridge offering clear knowledge of theory and practice to the literate but not Latinate surgeon. On the other hand, not all surgeons (or physicians or apothecaries) went through the process of applying to the Protomedicato for a license. Indeed, the constant tensions and disputes between various municipal leaders and crown officials created many opportunities for medical practitioners to find support and acceptance within local jurisdictions without having to meet the increasingly stringent royal criteria. It is therefore also possible to see learned vernacular surgical texts as potentially undermining those royal regulations, providing up-to-date knowledge to those without a university education and therefore enabling them to sharpen their knowledge and skills without meeting royal educational criteria. The question of both their intention and their effect—whether they acted in support of or in opposition to the royal mandates—is just one of the reasons these surgeons remain so intriguing.

The Médico y Cirujano

In the opening book of his *Cirugía universal*, Juan Calvo addresses the learned surgeon specifically, referring repeatedly to "el Médico y Cirujano"—that is to say, *the* physician-surgeon, rather than physicians and surgeons. Citing Hippocrates, he briefly recounts cases when they may not succeed in healing: some ailments are immediately mortal, such as wounds to the heart or apoplexy (sudden death with no apparent external reason); some ailments are not necessarily mortal but become so through the actions of the patient; some will become mortal days after the patient appears to recover well. Calvo aims to reassure against such problems, asserting that "it is sufficient that the Médico y Cirujano rationally and carefully apply the proper remedies for the condition" even if, in the end, it does not save the patient.[65] In this way, Calvo subtly moves the learned surgeon out of the ancient view of surgery as a set of manual skills with generally clear success when applied properly, and into the view of medicine (physic) in which forces are at work in the body that may not be visible or controllable. In embracing the theoretical aspects of medicine, surgeons must be willing to embrace uncertainty. It was a trade-off many seem to have been willing to make.

In Spain, surgical practitioners were generally divided into three categories, referring to their education and training: Latin, *romancista*, and specialist.[66] At the top of the system (the highest in social status) were the Latin surgeons (*cirujanos latinos*), so-called because of their higher education, signified by knowledge of Latin. Below them were the *cirujanos romancistas*: literate, licensed (by guild, apprenticeship, municipality, or another group), and well-trained but lacking knowledge of Latin or a university degree. Trained by apprenticeship, which often began around age fourteen, these surgeons made up the bulk of surgical practitioners in cities and towns across Spain. We generally know little about them, for they did not keep case records and did not publish other kinds of texts. Many *romancistas* were certainly literate, as shown by the wealth of vernacular medical texts circulating, as well as occasional postmortem inventories that include books, although often relatively few in number.[67] Much more work is needed to uncover the roles they played in society and how the intellectual and social changes described in this book affected them. The third category of practitioners were the specialists who may have learned by apprenticeship and then honed their skills by experience. They generally provided limited services focused usually on just one or two physical complaints, such as cataracts, hernia, broken bones, or dental problems.

The men at the center of this study were *cirujanos latinos*, a small group of elite and highly educated surgeons. They all studied at universities in Spain, and though they were not all of the same generation, all were practicing before the 1560s when surgical courses began to be taught in universities. It is not clear that all held full medical degrees, but they seem to have at least an arts degree and a good working knowledge of Latin (and perhaps some Greek medical terminology). Two of them wrote texts in Latin, and those who wrote in the vernacular were careful to justify this as a choice not a necessity. Often calling themselves médico y cirujano to denote their medical along with surgical training, they were in many cases equal in status (and sometimes income) to physicians.[68]

The term *médico* was a general one, so those who used it could also use either the title of *doctor* to denote a full doctoral degree from a university (which like today was a title used by medical doctors, as well as doctors of theology or law) or *licenciado*, which could denote either a university degree or could indicate a form of royal licensing. This dual title of médico y cirujano was variable in its use. Used frequently by the practitioners themselves in their texts and in municipal records, it does not appear in other official records. For example, Francisco Díaz, styles himself "médico y chyrujano de la C.R.M. del Rey don Phelippe nuestro Señor y doctor y maestro en hpilosophia [sic]" on the title page of his 1575 surgical text. His subsequent 1588 treatise on urology refers to him as "Dotor en medicina, y maestro en filosofia, por la insigne universidad de Alcala de Henares, y Cirujano del Rey, nuestro Señor." The first title attaches the expertise of the surgeon to him at the outset, while the second acknowledges it only at the end. Madrid parish records of baptism for his children refer to him as "doctor," while the official records from the royal court of his position award him "Titulo de Cirujano de la Casa Real."[69]

Learned surgeons, by whatever titles they were known, appear frequently by the mid-sixteenth century. Their comprehensive texts, published (and often republished) in the last decades of the century, are the most prominent records they left, but they could be found working in cities across the peninsula. They were the products of a long complex tradition of surgical education, training, and regulation. Their appearance and our ability to understand them are due in no small part to the expansion of the printing press, which encouraged intellectuals in many fields to codify and record their knowledge. In the case of these surgeons, their knowledge resonated a remarkably long time so that translations and further reprintings through the next century further ensured their lasting impact.

Notes

1 Faith Wallis, "Pre-Modern Surgery: Wounds, Words, and the Paradox of 'Tradition,'" in *The Palgrave Handbook of the History of Surgery*, ed. Thomas Schlich (London: Palgrave Macmillan, 2018), 52–6; Mathias Witt, "Surgery," in *The Cambridge Companion to Hippocrates*, ed. Peter E. Pormann (New York: Cambridge University Press, 2018), 217–19; D. W. Amundsen, "Medicine and Surgery as Art or Craft: The Role of Schematic Literature in the Separation of Medicine and Surgery in the Late Middle Ages," *Transactions & Studies of the College of Physicians of Philadelphia*, 5, no. 1 (1979): 43–6.

2 Witt, "Surgery," 218–19.

3 Celsus, *De Medicina*, trans. W. G. Spencer (Perseus Digital Library), bks. 1, Prooemium, accessed October 16, 2021, http://www.perseus.tufts.edu/hopper/text?doc=urn:cts:latinLit:phi0836.phi002.perseus-eng1:1.pr.

4 Wallis, "Pre-Modern Surgery: Wounds, Words, and the Paradox of 'Tradition,'" 55.

5 E. Savage-Smith, "The Practice of Surgery in Islamic Lands: Myth and Reality," *Social History of Medicine* 13, no. 2 (2000): 307–21, https://doi.org/10.1093/shm/13.2.307.

6 Monica H. Green and Brian Long, "Ego Constantinus Africanus Montis Cassinensis Monacus," *Constantinus Africanus* (blog), n.d., https://constantinusafricanus.com/; Monica Helen Green, ed., *The Trotula: A Medieval Compendium of Women's Medicine* (Philadelphia: University of Pennsylvania Press, 2001).

7 Nancy G. Siraisi, *Medieval & Early Renaissance Medicine: An Introduction to Knowledge and Practice* (Chicago: University of Chicago Press, 1990), 70–7.

8 Jon Arrizabalaga, "Spanish Medical Students' Peregrinato to Italian Universities in the Renaissance," in *Centres of Medical Excellence? Medical Travel and Education in Europe 1500–1789*, ed. Ole Peter Grell, Andrew Cunningham, and Jon Arrizabalaga (Burlington, VT: Ashgate, 2010), 93–4; Luca Mattei, "Estudio de la Madraza de Granada a partir del registro arqueológico y de las metodologías utilizadas en la intervención del 2006," *Arqueología y Territorio*, no. 5 (2008): 182–3.

9 Luis García Ballester, "Medical Science and Medical Teachings at the University of Salamanca in the 15th Century," in *Universities and Science in the Early Modern Period*, ed. Mordechai Feingold and Víctor Navarro Brotons, Archimedes, v. 12 (Dordrecht: Springer, 2006), 38–9.

10 Michael McVaugh and Luis García Ballester, "The Medical Faculty at Early Fourteenth-Century Lérida," in *History of Universities*, ed. Laurence Brockliss, History of Universities 8 (Oxford: Oxford University Press, 1989), 2–3.

11 See, for example, Michael R. McVaugh, *Medicine before the Plague: Practitioners and Their Patients in the Crown of Aragon, 1285–1345* (Cambridge: Cambridge University Press, 2002), 78–9.
12 Scholars of medieval medicine, Michael McVaugh foremost among them, have illuminated and analyzed this early rational and text-based surgery. Michael McVaugh, "Surgical Education in the Middle Ages," *Dynamis: Acta Hispanica Ad Medicinae Scientiarumque Historiam Illustrandam* 20 (2000): 283–304; Michael R. McVaugh, *The Rational Surgery of the Middle Ages*, Micrologus' Library 15 (Firenze: SISMEL-Edizione del Galluzzo, 2006); Monica Green, "Crafting a (Written) Science of Surgery: The First European Surgical Texts," *REMEDIA* (blog), October 13, 2015, https://remedianetwork.net/2015/10/13/crafting-a-written-science-of-surgery-the-first-european-surgical-texts/; Nancy G. Siraisi, "How to Write a Latin Book on Surgery: Organizing Principles and Authorial Devices in Guglielmo Da Saliceto and Dino Del Garbo," in *Practical Medicine from Salerno to the Black Death*, ed. Luis García Ballester et al. (New York: Cambridge University Press, 1994), 88–109; Wallis, "Pre-Modern Surgery: Wounds, Words, and the Paradox of 'Tradition.'"
13 Michael McVaugh, "When Universities First Encountered Surgery," *Journal of the History of Medicine and Allied Sciences* 72, no. 1 (2017): 288–91; The *Estudi* was subsequently absorbed into the University of Valencia upon its founding in 1499. Bjørn Okholm Skaarup, *Anatomy and Anatomists in Early Modern Spain*, (Burlington, VT: Ashgate, 2015), 34; Laurence Brockliss and Colin Jones, *The Medical World of Early Modern France* (New York: Oxford University Press, 1997), 94.
14 McVaugh, *The Rational Surgery of the Middle Ages*, 41–4.
15 Katharine Park, "The Criminal and the Saintly Body: Autopsy and Dissection in Renaissance Italy," *Renaissance Quarterly* 47, no. 1 (1994): 4–7, https://doi.org/10.2307/2863109.
16 José M. López Piñero, "The Faculty of Medicine of Valencia," in *Universities and Science in the Early Modern Period*, ed. Mordechai Feingold and Víctor Navarro Brotons, Archimedes, v. 12 (Dordrecht: Springer, 2006), 65–82; Karen Reeds, *Botany in Medieval and Renaissance Universities*, Harvard Dissertations in the History of Science (New York: Garland, 1991).
17 Charles Donald O'Malley, *Andreas Vesalius of Brussels, 1514–1564* (Berkeley: University of California Press, 1965), 205–6; Jerome J. Bylebyl, "The School of Padua: Humanistic Medicine in the Sixteenth Century," in *Health, Medicine and Mortality in the Sixteenth Century*, ed. Charles Webster (New York: Cambridge University Press, 1979), 359–60.
18 Ian Maclean, *Logic, Signs and Nature in the Renaissance: The Case of Learned Medicine* (New York: Cambridge University Press, 2007), 20–2.
19 Vivian Nutton, "Humanist Surgery," in *The Medical Renaissance of the Sixteenth Century*, ed. A. Wear, R. K. French, and Iain M. Lonie (New York: Cambridge University Press, 2009), 75–99; Richard J. Durling, "A Chronological Census of Renaissance Editions and Translations of Galen," *Journal of the Warburg and Courtauld Institutes* 24, no. 3/4 (1961): 230, https://doi.org/10.2307/750797.
20 Maclean, *Logic, Signs and Nature in the Renaissance*, 21; Nancy G. Siraisi, "The Changing Fortunes of a Traditional Text: Goals and Strategies in Sixteenth-Century Latin Editions of the Canon of Avicenna," in *The Medical Renaissance of the Sixteenth Century*, ed. A. Wear, R. K. French, and Iain M. Lonie (New York: Cambridge University Press, 2009), 16–41; Brockliss and Jones, *The Medical World of Early Modern France*, 93–6.
21 Inmaculada Delgado Jara and Rosa M. Herrera García, "Humanidades y Humanistas en la Universidad de Salamanca del siglo XV," in *Salamanca y su universidad en el primer Renacimiento: Siglo XV*, Miscelanea Alfonso IX (Salamanca: Universidad de Salamanca, 2010), 37; José Ignacio Blanco Pérez, *Humanistas médicos en el Renacimiento vallisoletano* (Burgos: Universidad de Burgos, 1999); López Piñero, "The Faculty of Medicine of Valencia"; Ana Isabel Martín Ferreira, *El humanismo médico en la Universidad de Alcalá: siglo XVI* (Alcalá: Universidad de Alcalá, 1995); M. Jesús Pérez Ibáñez, *El humanismo médico del siglo XVI en la Universidad de Salamanca*, Serie Lingüística y Filología, no. 31 (Valladolid: Universidad de Valladolid, Secretariado de Publicaciones e Intercambio Científico, 1998).

22 Several surgical authors, including Juan Fragoso, Francisco Díaz, and Dionisio Daza Chacón, include lists of authorities cited at the beginning or end of their texts. For others, later scholars have analyzed their citations. See José Luis Fresquet Febrer, "La diversidad de mentalidades en la 'Cirugia' (1580) de Juan Calvo, a través del estudio de sus referencias," in *Estudios sobre la medicina y ciencia valencianas (siglos XVI–XIX)*, ed. M. José Báguena Cervellera et al. (Valencia: Universidad de Valencia, 1985), 71–89; Francisco Arceo de Fregenal, *Método verdadero de curar las heridas y otros preceptos de este arte: Método de curar las fiebres*, ed. Andrés Oyola Fabián and J. Cobos Bueno, Bibliotheca Montaniana 21 (Huelva: Universidad de Huelva, 2009), 42–3.
23 McVaugh, "Surgical Education in the Middle Ages," 293–300.
24 R. K French, "Berengario Da Carpi and the Use of Commentary in Anatomical Teaching," in *The Medical Renaissance of the Sixteenth Century*, ed. A. Wear, R. K. French, and Iain M. Lonie (New York: Cambridge University Press, 2009), 48.
25 Barbara S. Bowers, ed., *The Medieval Hospital and Medical Practice*, AVISTA Studies in the History of Medieval Technology, Science and Art, v. 3 (Burlington, VT: Ashgate, 2007).
26 Guy Beaujouan, "La medicina y la cirugía en el monasterio de Guadalupe," *Asclepio: Revista de Historia de La Medicina y de La Ciencia* 17 (1965): 157.
27 Luis García Ballester, *La búsqueda de la salud: Sanadores y enfermos en la España medieval*, Historia, Ciencia y Sociedad 321 (Barcelona: Ediciones Península, 2001), 398; Sebastián García, O.F.M., "Medicina y cirugía en los Reales Hospitales de Guadalupe," *Revista de Estudios Extremeños* 59, no. 1 (2003): 11–77.
28 García, O.F.M., "Medicina y Cirugía en los Reales Hospitales de Guadalupe," 67–9.
29 See, for example, Juan Ignacio Carmona García, *El Sistema de Hospitalidad Pública en la Sevilla del Antiguo Régimen* (Sevilla: Excma. Diputación Provincial de Sevilla, 1979), 39–60; An excellent study of Toledo's hospital for morbo gálico is Cristian Berco, *From Body to Community: Venereal Disease and Society in Baroque Spain* (Toronto: University of Toronto Press, 2016); For the French Disease in Italy, see Jon Arrizabalaga, John Henderson, and R. K French, *The Great Pox: The French Disease in Renaissance Europe* (New Haven, CT: Yale University Press, 1997), 145–233.
30 María Luz López Terrada, "Health Care and Poor Relief in the Crown of Aragon," in *Health Care and Poor Relief in Counter-Reformation Europe*, ed. Ole Peter Grell, Andrew Cunningham, and Jon Arrizabalaga (New York: Routledge, 1999), 177–200.
31 Teresa Huguet-Termes, "Madrid Hospitals and Welfare in the Context of the Hapsburg Empire," *Medical History. Supplement*, no. 29 (2009): 64–85; Michele L. Clouse, *Medicine, Government and Public Health in Philip II's Spain: Shared Interests, Competing Authorities* (Burlington, VT: Ashgate, 2011), 143–67; Jon Arrizabalaga, "Poor Relief in Counter-Reformation Castile: An Overview," in *Health Care and Poor Relief in Counter-Reformation Europe*, ed. Ole Peter Grell, Andrew Cunningham, and Jon Arrizabalaga (New York: Routledge, 1999), 151–76.
32 Juan Calvo, *Primera y segunda parte de la cirugia uniuersal y particular del cuerpo humano* (Madrid: Diego Flamenco, 1626), 558–9.
33 Dionisio Daza Chacón, *Practica y teorica de cirugía en romance y en latin* (Valladolid: en casa de Ana Velez, 1609), Prologo al Lector; For a short biographical sketch in English, see Charles Donald O'Malley, "Dionisio Daza Chacon," in *Medizingeschichte in Unserer Zeit. Festgabe Fur Edith Heischkel-Artelt Und Walter Artelt Zum 65. Geburtstag.*, ed. Hans-Heinz Eulner et al. (Stuttgart: Ferndinand Enke Verlag, 1971), 160–70.
34 Francisco Díaz, *Compendio de chirurgia: En el qual de trata de todas las cosas tocantes la theorica y pratica della* (Madrid, 1575), fols. 1v–2.
35 Luis García Ballester, Michael R. McVaugh, and Agustín Rubio, *Medical Licensing and Learning in Fourteenth-Century Valencia*, Transactions of the American Philosophical Society, v. 79, pt. 6 (Philadelphia: American Philosophical Society, 1989); Iona McCleery, "Medical Licensing in Late Medieval Portugal," in *Medicine and the Law in the Middle Ages*, ed. Wendy J. Turner and Sara M. Butler, Medieval Law and Its Practice, volume 17 (Leiden: Brill, 2014), 196–7; M. R. McVaugh, *Medicine before the Plague: Practitioners and Their Patients in the Crown of Aragon, 1285–1345* (New York: Cambridge University Press, 1993), 95–103.

36 Katharine Park, *Doctors and Medicine in Early Renaissance Florence* (Princeton, NJ: Princeton University Press, 1985); García Ballester, McVaugh, and Rubio, *Medical Licensing and Learning in Fourteenth-Century Valencia*; McCleery, "Medical Licensing in Late Medieval Portugal."
37 Brockliss and Jones, *The Medical World of Early Modern France*, 214–21; Mercedes Gallent Marco, "El Colegio de Barberos y Cirujanos de Valencia: Aportación Documental," *Saitabi: Revista de La Facultat de Geografia i Història* 43 (1993): 147–55; Asunción Fernández Doctor, "Médicos y cirujanos de Zaragoza en la edad moderna. Su número y estructura sociofamiliar," *Dynamis: Acta Hispanica Ad Medicinae Scientiarumque Historiam Illustrandam* 17 (1997): 143–4.
38 McVaugh, "Surgical Education in the Middle Ages," 293.
39 McVaugh, 293.
40 García Ballester, McVaugh, and Rubio, *Medical Licensing and Learning in Fourteenth-Century Valencia*, 2–10.
41 For a further discussion of the regional differences in regulatory systems and conflicts within them, see María Luz López Terrada, "The Control of Medical Practice Under the Spanish Monarchy During the Sixteenth and Seventeenth Centuries," in *Más allá de la Leyenda Negra: España y la Revolución Científica = Beyond the Black Legend: Spain and the Scientific Revolution*, ed. Víctor Navarro Brotons and William Eamon (Valencia: Univ. de València, Inst. de Historia de la Ciencia y Documentación López Piñero, 2007), 281–94.
42 Clouse, *Medicine, Government and Public Health in Philip II's Spain*, 16–17.
43 María Soledad Campos Díez, *El Real Tribunal del Protomedicato Castellano, Siglos XIV–XIX* (Cuenca: Ediciones de la Universidad de Castilla-La Mancha, 1999), 25–42; Clouse, *Medicine, Government and Public Health in Philip II's Spain*, 15–20.
44 María Soledad Campos Díez, "El Protomedicato en la administración central de la Monarquía Hispánica," *Dynamis: Acta Hispanica ad Medicinae Scientiarumque Historiam Illustrandam* 16 (1996): 48.
45 Clouse, *Medicine, Government and Public Health in Philip II's Spain*, 19–22.
46 Details of many of these smaller changes and the debates surrounding them may be found in Miguel Eugenio Muñoz, *Recopilación de las leyes, pragmaticas reales, decretos, y acuerdos del Real Tribunal del Proto-Medicato* (Valencia: En la Imprenta de la viuda de Antonio Bordazar, 1751).
47 Clouse, *Medicine, Government and Public Health in Philip II's Spain*, 25–6.
48 David C. Goodman, *Power and Penury: Government, Technology, and Science in Philip II's Spain* (New York: Cambridge University Press, 1988), 222–3.
49 Clouse, *Medicine, Government and Public Health in Philip II's Spain*, 22–4.
50 Bjørn Okholm Skaarup, *Anatomy and Anatomists in Early Modern Spain*, History of Medicine in Context (Burlington, VT: Ashgate, 2015), 34.
51 Luis García Ballester, "La cirugía en la Valencia del siglo XV. El privilegio de desecar cadaveres en 1477," *Cuadernos de Historia de La Medicina Española* 7 (1967): 155–76.
52 Skaarup, *Anatomy and Anatomists in Early Modern Spain*, 68–75, 116–22.
53 Clouse, *Medicine, Government and Public Health in Philip II's Spain*, 46–7.
54 Clouse, 56; Skaarup, *Anatomy and Anatomists in Early Modern Spain*, 114.
55 María Luz López Terrada, "Medical Pluralism in the Iberian Kingdoms: The Control of Extra-academic Practitioners in Valencia," *Medical History Supplement* 29 (2009): 8–9; López Terrada, "The Control of Medical Practice Under the Spanish Monarchy During the Sixteenth and Seventeenth Centuries."
56 Martin Biersack, "The Adoption of Humanism in Catholic Spain (1470–1520)," *Reformation & Renaissance Review* 21, no. 1 (2019): 27–46, https://doi.org/10.1080/14622459.2019.1568371; Susan Byrne, *Ficino in Spain* (Toronto: University of Toronto Press, 2015); Lu Ann Homza, "Erasmus as Hero, or Heretic? Spanish Humanism and the Valladolid Assembly of 1527," *Renaissance Quarterly* 50, no. 1 (1997): 78–118, https://doi.org/10.2307/3039329.
57 Henry Kamen, *The Spanish Inquisition: A Historical Revision* (New Haven, CT: Yale University Press, 1998), 103–8.

58 Víctor Navarro Brotons and William Eamon, eds., *Más allá de la Leyenda Negra: España y la Revolución Científica = Beyond the Black Legend: Spain and the Scientific Revolution* (Valencia: Univ. de València, Inst. de Historia de la Ciencia y Documentación López Piñero, 2007) The preface summarizes the older scholarship. The included essays represent many of the scholars who have collectively revised the view of Spanish scientific scholarship.
59 See, for example, Alejandro Coroleu, "Humanismo en España," in *Introducción al Humanismo Renacentista*, ed. Jill Kraye (Cambridge: Cambridge University Press, 1998), 295–330; Josep Lluís Barona and Xavier Gómez Font, *La correspondencia de Carolus Clusius con los científicos españoles* (València: Universitat de València, 1998); María M. Portuondo, *The Spanish Disquiet: The Biblical Natural Philosophy of Benito Arias Montano* (Chicago: The University of Chicago Press, 2019); Enrique Martínez Ruiz and José María López Piñero, eds., *Felipe II, la ciencia y la técnica* (Madrid: Actas Editorial, 1999); Navarro Brotons and Eamon, *Más allá de la Leyenda Negra.*
60 See, for example, Skaarup's work on anatomical study in Spain: Skaarup, *Anatomy and Anatomists in Early Modern Spain.*
61 Luis S. Granjel, *La Medicina Española Renacentista*, Historia General de La Medicina Española, II (Salamanca: Universidad de Salamanca, 1980), 15; Clouse, *Medicine, Government and Public Health in Philip II's Spain*, 62.
62 Clouse, *Medicine, Government and Public Health in Philip II's Spain*, 47.
63 Campos Díez, *El Real Tribunal del Protomedicato Castellano, Siglos XIV–XIX*, 72–84; Luis Martín Santos, *Barberos y cirujanos de los siglos XVI y XVII* (Valladolid: Junta de Castilla y León, Consejería de Educación y Cultura, 2000), 11–13.
64 Clouse, *Medicine, Government and Public Health in Philip II's Spain*, 61.
65 Calvo, *Cirugia uniuersal*, 2.
66 See the discussion in María Luz López Terrada, "Médicos, Cirujanos, Boticarios y Albéitares," in *Historia de La Ciencia y de La Técnica En La Corona de Castilla*, ed. José María López Piñero, vol. III (Valladolid: Junta de Castilla y León, Consejería de Educación y Cultura, 2002), 168–74.
67 See, for example, Anastasio Rojo Vega, *Enfermos y sanadores en la Castilla del siglo XVI*, Historia y sociedad 34 (Valladolid: Universidad de Valladolid, 1993), 33–6.
68 José María López Piñero, *Ciencia y técnica en la sociedad española de los siglos XVI y XVII* (Barcelona: Labor Universitaria, 1979), 83.
69 Mercedes Agulló y Cobo, *Documentos sobre médicos españoles de los siglos XVI al XVIII*, vol. XII, Cuadernos de Historia de La Medicina Española (Salamanca: Universidad de Salamanca, 1969), 33; Juan Manuel Jiménez Muñoz, *Médicos y cirujanos en "Quitaciones de Corte" (1435–1715)* (Valladolid: Universidad de Valladolid, 1977), 37–8.

2

SPANISH LEARNED SURGEONS

A Broad and Connected Movement

In the fourth book of his *Cirugía universal*, Juan Calvo addresses the question of how to treat nerves that have been severed. He begins by acknowledging this was a matter of great debate. On the side that argued such nerves cannot be repaired or regrown, he cites several earlier medieval authorities and, "among the moderns Fragoso in his Gloss, and Dionisio de Daza in the second part of Wounds chapter 59." After discussing this view in some detail, he turns to the other side, those who argue that nerves could be at least reattached, again referencing several authorities "and among the moderns Alcaçar, discussing nerve wounds in chapter 14."[1] In this one short passage, Calvo demonstrates his integration within an intellectual network of his colleagues. Calvo had no personal connection to the men he cites, though Fragoso and Daza Chacón may have known one another as both served members of the royal family. Despite his lack of personal ties, Calvo knew their work well and knew that their inclusion in this passage would signal to readers his participation in an ongoing conversation. Juan Fragoso, whose text predated that of Calvo, includes fewer references to contemporary surgeons in his discussion of severed nerves, but just a few pages earlier in discussing a separate question of when to remove an embedded weapon from a wound, he offers a series of case studies or stories he has read or heard from fellow surgeons. Several of these are unnamed sources, given in the text as simply "a modern author," "a story of another noble," "a doctor recounted to me."[2] Similar small references are sprinkled throughout all learned surgical texts, a constant reminder that these men were not simply individual practitioners but were also part of a larger community of men, ideas, and practices.

Scholars have long recognized the importance of connections between early modern scientists in intellectual networks that often reached across geographic, linguistic, and religious boundaries. Among the best known of these were the correspondence networks such as those of Carolus Clusius, Nicolas Pieresc, and Henry

DOI: 10.4324/9781003291060-3

Oldenham.[3] Other scholars have utilized Jesuit correspondence to show an internal network that also circulated scientific and medical information across distances.[4] But networks were also formed in more indirect ways, such as through studying or working in the same city, patronage networks, and the circulation of printed texts.[5] Networks were most often supportive groups, exchanging and circulating both ideas and material goods, but they could also foster disagreements. As the example of Calvo shows, printing facilitated the rapid and wide circulation of ideas among intellectuals who did not know each other personally, which in turn could enable not only the formation of new connections but also the eruption and expansion of intellectual disputes.

Spanish Renaissance surgeons formed a loose collection of practitioners and scholars in several of these indirect ways. They were both local practitioners and national rivals, as well as colleagues, defenders, and detractors of each other. They were influential not only as university professors, court practitioners, and Protomédicos in their own lifetimes but also as authors of authoritative texts that continued to be reprinted and studied for the next century. Several had their works translated and disseminated across Europe as well. They were connected in a variety of ways, some by where they practiced (at court or in various cities), others through mutual friends, and some by reading and responding to each other's work, both favorably and unfavorably. They did not merely coexist in the same era, they responded to, assisted, and challenged one another. These overlapping circles of interaction are a key part of why historians have so often treated them as a group.[6] Their interactions—not only in working alongside each other and citing each other's work but also in debates over theory and practice—are an important window into the intellectual vitality of the era.

Brief biographies of each of the surgeons discussed in the book are provided in the appendix. Some of them, such as Antonio Pérez, we know very little about, while others, such as Dionisio Daza Chacón, appear in many different records and shared a great deal of their own biographical information in their texts. Here they will be generally introduced by examining both the connections between them and the diversity among them. One of the things that makes this surgical renaissance so striking is the great diversity of men who participated in it, both geographic and intellectual. Within Spain, learned surgeons studied at various institutions with medical faculties: Salamanca, Valladolid, Alcalá de Henares, and Valencia. From these educational centers, graduates dispersed across both Castile and Aragon to gain practical experience and begin their careers. Andrés de León, for example, studied in Seville but also trained in surgery at hospitals in Zaragoza and Valencia. Juan Calvo studied in Valencia and then gained further training at the General Hospital in Zaragoza. Fragoso studied in Alcalá de Henares, then practiced in Seville before moving to the court in Madrid. Their career paths were quite varied, as some learned surgeons were employed by city or town officials at hospitals, jails, and Inquisition offices, while others worked in private employment in the service of nobles or as independent practitioners. On average they each published two to three texts, with at least one reprinting. Some, like Juan Fragoso, published several texts (Fragoso published five), while others, such as Francisco Arceo, published only one. Three principal things unite them: they were university educated, actively practiced surgery in the same era (roughly 1550–1605), and published learned texts that were influential.

The learned surgeons at the heart of this study did not all know each other directly, yet the contextual connections between them are strong. Some of the connections discussed here are modern impositions of order, such as grouping them by age, intended audience, or career path. Other connections, however, were more directly personal to them as they crossed paths living and working in the same places and responded to one another's ideas. To begin with, we can divide them into two generations, as López Piñero did in his seminal study.[7] An older generation, born around the turn of the sixteenth century (Andrés Alcázar, Francisco Arceo, and Dionisio Daza Chacón) and a second generation, born in the 1530s (Juan Calvo, Juan Fragoso, Francisco Díaz, Bartolomé Hidalgo de Agüero, Antonio Pérez, Andrés de León). The last two, Antonio Pérez and Andrés de León, we have the least information about. They were likely born in the 1530s, though perhaps up to a decade later, given their presumed deaths sometime in the early seventeenth century. These groupings by age make little difference when we look at their writings, however, for despite the thirty-year gap between them, all published within the same time frame of 1565–1605.

A second informal division emerges when we look at their intended audiences, dividing them into those who wrote in Latin (Francisco Arceo and Andrés Alcázar) and those who wrote in the vernacular (all the others). While Dionisio Daza Chacón's full surgical work, *Practica y theorica de cirugia en romance y latin* (1585) promised both Castilian and Latin, the text was in Castilian with references to Latin texts. Juan Fragoso is an exception in that he wrote works on materia medica in Latin but works on surgery in Castilian. The choice to write in Latin or the vernacular gives us some insight into the internal disputes of the surgical renaissance, particularly who should benefit from access to the combination of classical knowledge and innovative practices they offered. While the Latin authors insisted that they were raising the status of surgical knowledge by restricting access only to those properly educated and able to read Latin, vernacular authors expressed a desire to raise the status of surgery by raising the skill and knowledge level of current practitioners who may not have had the opportunity of Latin study but were dedicated to their craft nonetheless. Francisco Arceo and Andrés Alcázar, the two who held firmly to Latin, were also among the earliest of this group to publish (1574 and 1575), so their texts were widely studied, disputed, and cited by the later surgical authors who wrote in the vernacular.

We find a wider diversity among them in the range of specialized interests they pursued. Most of these learned surgeons wrote late in life, after decades of experience. Their work and interests diverged, making their texts unique reflections of their personalities. While Juan Calvo, Juan Fragoso, and Dionisio Daza Chacón wrote comprehensive treatises (covering anatomy, wounds, fractures, abscesses, ulcers, and so forth), others focused more narrowly, such as Bartolomé Hidalgo de Agüero on a particular method of healing wounds, Francisco Arceo and Andrés Alcázar on head wounds, and Francisco Díaz on urology. Several of them also wrote separate texts or short treatises within their larger surgical texts on specific diseases, particularly plague and morbo gálico. Hidalgo de Agüero also wrote an early treatise on typhus, while Juan Fragoso was unique in writing his three texts on materia medica.[8]

Finally, the divisions and connections between these men also become apparent when we group them by career path: those who practiced at court (Juan Fragoso and Francisco Díaz), those who served the crown in military service (Dionisio Daza Chacón, Antonio Pérez, Andrés de León), and those who taught, whether associated with a university (Andrés Alcázar, Juan Calvo, Bartolomé Hidalgo de Agüero) or privately (Francisco Arceo). Their varied paths brought many of these men into contact with one another, but the myriad differences in careers are equally important. They demonstrate the wide-ranging nature of the surgical renaissance and its proponents. One figure did not lead the way, one career path did not provide greater prominence, and one aspect of surgical practice did not gain greater public recognition. Instead, the surgical renaissance crossed boundaries of language, geography, training, and specialized interests.

Royal Service

Court Surgeons

The largest subset of learned surgeons were those associated with royal service, both as personal practitioners for the royal family and military surgeons in service to members of the royal family or other nobles. The court remained the most important site for patronage of learned surgeons, as was the case across all European territories. Most of the best-known figures of sixteenth-century surgery were enabled by and are remembered for their high-level patrons, such as Pierre Franco and Ambroise Paré at the court of Henri II, Giovanni da Vigo at the court of Pope Julius II, Thomas Vicary at Henry VIII's court, and, of course, Andreas Vesalius, who gained the patronage of Emperor Charles V and then remained in the employ of Philip II of Spain.

Charles V's patronage of Vesalius brought the renowned anatomist to his court, where he joined the learned surgeon Dionisio Daza Chacón and others serving the emperor during the Hapsburg-Valois Wars (1521–59). These and other concerns kept Charles out of Spain more often than not, and therefore much of the task of ruling in Spain fell to his son, Philip, once he was of age to act as regent. The regionalism of Spain meant the court had a long tradition of mobility, and it was not until mid-century that Philip II rooted the court in Madrid. Even so, Philip continued to travel frequently, visiting different parts of his Iberian realm and residing for stretches at other residences such as Aranjuez, located just south of Madrid, and El Escorial, the monastery and royal residence he built to commemorate the victory of Spanish forces against the French at Saint-Quentin in 1557. Indeed, according to

Geoffrey Parker, Philip "spent less than half his life" in Madrid, though his court surgeons and physicians would not have always traveled with him, particularly when he sought retreat from the stresses of rule.[9] Thus, by the later sixteenth century, Madrid was the administrative center of the Spanish court, even when the king was away. As a result, the town, and more specifically the royal court, became an important intellectual and cultural center, as well as a center of nobility and patronage whose fortunes were tied to the fortunes of the monarchy itself. A court appointment was the highest patronage one could achieve in this era. It was reward or recognition for achievements, as well as a result of working through lower-level patronage networks, but also served as an important platform from which to gain wider recognition, especially by publishing. Thus, for some, such as Juan Fragoso, the invitation to join the royal court came because of their work and publications, while others, such as Dionisio Daza Chacón, used their experiences at court to shape their public outreach. Fragoso had practiced for a decade and already published two works when elevated to a position at court, while Daza Chacón did not publish until after his retirement at (approximately) age 70. In his preface, Daza Chacón explicitly refers to his experience having served on the Protomedicato examining surgeons as part of his motivation in writing. In addition, Daza Chacón is highly retrospective in his text, offering experiences as part of his explanation and justification for the debates he weighs in on (such as how to treat gunshot wounds) and the innovations he presents (how to clip aneurysms, how to ligate arteries in limb amputations, a method for removing nasal polyps). He was not the first to write on these, the French surgeon Ambroise Paré had made his career (and lasting fame) by writing about them decades before. It was not priority recognition that Daza Chacón sought, it was correct and useful knowledge, both theoretical and practical.

While Dionisio Daza Chacón entered royal service under Charles V, it was during the reign of his son, Philip II, that learned surgeons flourished in Spain. Philip II maintained a strong interest in both science and medicine, and his court attracted a wide range of knowledgeable practitioners of both, holding varied educational backgrounds, from across Europe.[10] Philip's particular interest in maintaining large numbers of medical consultants is often attributed to his experiences of poor health, both his own and that of family members. In addition to periodic illnesses, such as fevers, colds, and stomach problems, Philip's chronic conditions included gallstones, malaria, and gout.[11] He outlived all four of his wives, two of whom died from complications in childbirth (María of Portugal in 1545 and Isabel of Valois in 1568), one from cancer (Mary Tudor in 1558), and the last, Anna of Austria, during an influenza epidemic (1580).[12] Like many of the era, Philip also lost five of his eight children at varying ages. He was known to make disparaging remarks about doctors, no doubt a reflection of his dependence upon them, famously proclaiming, in one of his sour moods that "physicians are terrible people."[13] He employed quite a lot of them, though, increasing the number of medical practitioners at court from the average of twenty employed by his father, Charles V, to a high of forty-seven in the early 1580s.[14] At least part of this increase, it should be noted, seems to have been a result of maintaining medical professionals at his favored alternate residence, El

Escorial, as well as those in Madrid.[15] Several of Philip II's royal physicians were very prominent and influential practitioners, including Luís Mercado (1525–1611), Francisco Valles (1524–92), and Cristóbal de Vega (1510–c.1573).[16]

In addition to his retinue of regular physicians and surgeons, Philip II also supported the work of several medical innovators. As Michele Clouse's work has demonstrated, Philip took a particular interest in investigating and supporting the work of empirics, particularly when they promised new healing methods.[17] These empirics, some formally educated and some only trained through apprenticeship, varied in their specialties, treating urinary stones, hernias, and broken bones, among other things. The Italian healer, alchemist, author, and professor of secrets Leonardo Fioravanti (1518–88) spent roughly a year at the court in Madrid (1576–7) before running afoul of the Protomedicato for practicing without a license and other charges. He followed in the metaphoric footsteps of Alfonso Díaz (d. 1567) who arrived from Rome (and became known in Spain as "Dr. Romano") with a method of curing urinary strictures, and the Spaniard Aparicio de Zubia (d. 1566), an empiric whose famous healing oil brought him royal support from both Charles V and Philip II, as well as international recognition.[18]

Along with these various empirics, Philip II also supported the new learned surgery and those who practiced and wrote about it. He employed university-educated surgeons to serve himself and his family and approved for publication (through his proxies at the Protomedicato), the publication of all of their texts. Among the many practitioners employed at court were two of the surgeons under consideration here, Juan Fragoso and Francisco Díaz.

Juan Fragoso began his career in Seville in the 1550s, where he was a part of the city's intellectual network, discussed in more detail later in this chapter. He became good friends with Francisco Hernández, a fellow graduate in medicine from the University of Alcalá de Henares, though Hernández had graduated years before Fragoso. The two shared an interest in medical botany and spent time together exploring the local region for materia medica. Both moved into royal service about a decade later, Hernández first around 1560 as a royal physician and later appointed as Protomédico de las Indias. His royal mandate included compiling information on the flora and fauna of both New Spain and Peru, a task for which he spent seven years working and studying in New Spain.[19] Fragoso followed him to court by 1566, first as a surgeon in the household of Queen Isabel (Elizabeth) of Valois and then transferring to Philip's service following her death in 1568.[20] His interest in botany also continued, and in addition to his surgical texts, he published three well-known texts on materia medica, all of which underwent reprinting for many years. The first was a Latin catalogue of medicinal simples, the *Catalogus simplicium medicamentorum* in 1566; the second a 1572 vernacular treatise on foreign materia medica, *Discurso de las cosas aromáticas* based on the work of the Portuguese physician Garcia d'Orta in India (though without crediting him); and the third, another Latin work, *De succedaneis medicamentis*, published in 1575. His surgical writing, meanwhile, began in 1570 with *Erotemas chirurgicas*, followed by the first edition of what became the *Cirugía universal* in 1573. This last text Fragoso continued to update and expand over the subsequent decades until his death in 1597, publishing at least six different editions in Madrid.[21]All of these works proved extremely popular and were reprinted frequently. The *Discursos de la cosas aromaticas* was translated into Latin and printed in Strasbourg several times in the seventeenth century (1600, 1601, 1639). His surgical work saw at least eleven reprintings in the seventeenth century, several of which were editions by Gerónimo de Ayala, who combined Fragoso's surgical work with an anatomical study by Francisco Núñez (1683, 1693, 1705, 1716, 1724).[22] An Italian translation of part of Fragoso's surgical work was printed in Palermo in 1639 and Venice in 1662 and 1686. In addition, Fragoso's books circulated widely across the Atlantic, appearing throughout the New World in libraries and inventories.[23]

Among other things, Fragoso is often remembered for his public dispute with Bartolomé Hidalgo de Agüero over wound treatment. The parameters and issues at stake in this dispute are addressed in detail in the next chapter, but it is worth pointing out here that the two men led virtually parallel lives, born almost at the same time and dying in the same year. Both were also connected to Seville and the intellectual circle that emerged there in the second half of the sixteenth century, and both wrote texts that were enormously influential, undergoing various reprintings into the next century and found in libraries not only in Spain but across the Atlantic as well.[24]

The second court surgeon, Francisco Díaz, provides an interesting contrast to Fragoso in both his background and professional interests. He gained his position at court at roughly the same time as Fragoso, the late 1560s, but came to it seeking a fresh start after years of practice in Burgos.

In 1557, shortly after finishing the last of his degrees, Díaz was one of sixteen applicants who underwent a public exam for an open position at the royal Hospital de la Corte in Valladolid. Here he crossed paths with Dionisio Daza Chacón, another learned surgeon whose life and career are discussed later in this chapter. Daza Chacón won the position at the Hospital, and Díaz relocated to Burgos, but his strong performance at this exam may have stood him in good purpose a decade later when he returned seeking, and ultimately receiving, a position at court.

In 1564–5, he lost his wife and daughter during a plague epidemic and so returned to his hometown of Alcalá with his surviving five children to be closer to his family.[25] He soon remarried and a few years later sought a position at court, which he achieved in 1570. Díaz was highly educated, with multiple degrees from the University of Alcalá de Henares, including bachelor of arts (1548), bachelor of medicine (1551), doctor of medicine (1555), and master of philosophy (1556). His intellectual interests ranged widely, as shown in his book collection, which included medicine, surgery, poetry, and philosophy in Spanish, Latin, and Greek. He was connected to the greatest writers of his time, including the famed playwright, novelist, and poet Lope de Vega, who wrote two sonnets for the preface to Díaz's book on urology, and Miguel de Cervantes, with whom he was friends by family connections and who refers to Díaz by name in *La Galatea*.[26]

Once at court, Díaz first published a treatise of surgery, *Compendio de chirurgia*, in 1575 and then one on urology, *Tratado nuevamente impresso, de todas las enfermedades de los riñones, vexiga, y carnosidades de la verga, y urina, dividido en tres libros*, in 1588. This latter text is what brought Díaz lasting fame. As the first complete text on urological problems and treatments, this was a result of his years of practice and an embrace of empiricism that enabled him to learn and then refine new techniques. Díaz himself credited the empiric Dr. Romano, mentioned earlier, from whom Díaz learned a method of treating blockages of the urethra. Díaz then added his own experiences and expertise in designing new instruments for this treatment. His work and text were foundational for establishing urology not just as an area of surgical expertise but also as a medical field in general.

Life at court gave both Fragoso and Díaz exposure to new ideas, opportunities to practice their craft, and time to refine their knowledge. Despite their differences in experiences and subspecialties, the two court surgeons remained tied together long after their deaths, as Fragoso's *Cirugia universal* and Díaz's *Tratado* on urology were reprinted together several times through the first half of the seventeenth century (1627, 1643, 1666).[27]

Military Surgeons

The second important group of learned royal surgeons were the military surgeons, Dionisio Daza Chacón, Antonio Pérez, and Andrés de León. While there is little direct evidence to personally connect these three men, their careers were strikingly intertwined in time and place. Daza Chacón, the oldest of them, remained the best known through later centuries, probably in part because he began his royal service under Charles V in the Hapsburg-Valois wars in Flanders in the 1540s, working on the battlefields alongside the more famous anatomist Andreas Vesalius. As a result of both Daza Chacón and Vesalius remaining in royal service under Philip II, they again collaborated (along with other medical experts) on two very famous cases of head wounds, that of King Henry II of France in 1559 and that of Philip II's son and heir, Don Carlos, in 1562. In the first case, the collected medical minds of France and Spain were unable to save the king from death, while the second case was resolved much more favorably under a collection of Spanish physicians and surgeons.[28] While many modern accounts overlook the contributions of Daza Chacón in these cases, his inclusion in both helped establish his presence as one of the foremost learned surgeons of his time. Daza Chacón's lengthy career and the trust he earned from Charles V and Philip II placed him as a participant in multiple international events of his time.

Dionisio Daza Chacón began his military career in 1543, serving the nobleman Don Pedro de Guzmán in Flanders. He quickly came to the attention of Charles V and joined the emperor's service shortly after. Decades later, after working in the households of various members of the royal family and at the Hospital de la Corte in Valladolid, his career became entwined with both Antonio Pérez and Andrés de León at the Rebellion of the Alpujarras (or Morisco Revolt) in 1569. Muslim residents of the remnant Kingdom of Granada, conquered in 1492 by Fernando and Isabel, had been forced to convert to Christianity at the turn of the century, creating the population of Moriscos, a term used to refer to both converts and their descendants. Increasing restrictions on that Morisco population over the next sixty years led eventually to a violent uprising named for the Alpujarras region of the Sierra Nevada mountains in which rebels were able to hold out against royal forces. The revolt broke out at the end of 1568. After a year of fighting, Philip II replaced the nobleman leading the response with his own half brother (Charles V's illegitimate son), Don Juan de Austria. It was among the forces that Don Juan brought to Granada that all three military surgeons were first brought together.

We know much less of the biographies of Pérez and León than that of Daza Chacón, and even the details of their military service are likewise much less clear. Andrés de León was from Granada and studied at the University of Seville. He then gained practical training working in the city alongside the famous physician Nicolas Monardes.[29] Monardes is best remembered for his multipart treatise on New World materia medica, which introduced Europeans to new medicinal plants, including tobacco, chocolate, and sassafras.[30] Working in Seville put León (along with Juan Fragoso mentioned earlier) in the ambit of a significant medical intellectual circle. In his surgical text, León also mentions practicing for a time at the Hospital del Cardenal in Seville, which possibly would have put him working under Bartolomé Hidalgo de Agüero, the head surgeon there, but we have no firm dates of when Hidalgo de Agüero began his tenure nor of when León was studying there. León's connections to any of those in the Seville circle remain vague, however, as it is unclear how long he was there before he moved on, also spending time working in hospitals in Valencia and Zaragoza. He then appears in royal military service by 1569 in the forces serving under Don Juan de Austria. This brought him geographically full circle back to Granada and into probable contact with Daza Chacón and Pérez, but he did not remain there long. Following the conclusion of the Rebellion of the Alpujarras, military service then took León from Andalucía northwards to the monastery of San Lorenzo de El Escorial as part of the retinue accompanying the translation of the royal remains of Emperor Charles V and Empress Isabel to the new royal mausoleum Philip II had built there. After some years at court, Léon ventured once again, this time to Portugal in the service of the Duke of Alba in 1580 for Philip II's conquest there. Nearly a decade later, he served as Protomédico and "médico y cirujano mayor" in the Armada sent against Queen Elizabeth in 1588.[31]

The background of our third military surgeon, Antonio Pérez, is even less clear, though we know that he was Portuguese and that he published his first book, *Summa y examen de cirugia*, one of the earliest learned vernacular surgical texts in Spain, in 1568. Tracing his biography is further complicated by the fact that Philip II employed a secretary of the same name, who remains much more famous as a result of his role in the scandalous 1578 murder of Juan de Escobedo, a secretary of Don Juan de Austria. For various reasons, Secretary Peréz remained a problematic focus of political attention and rumor for the rest of Philip's reign, from his arrest a decade after the event, to his escape from prison in 1590 and public accusations against the king as complicit in the murder.[32] In an ironic parallel, the surgeon Pérez was serving under Don Juan in the Netherlands even as Secretary Pérez enacted the assassination of Don Juan's secretary Escobedo.

What we can piece together of the military career of the surgeon Antonio Pérez begins, again, at the Rebellion of the Alpujarras. Following the settlement of the revolt in 1571, as Andrés de León remained in Spain, both Antonio Pérez and Dionisio Daza Chacón followed Don Juan de Austria to the Mediterranean, where the latter had been appointed to lead the fleet of the Holy League, an alliance of Catholic states fighting the Ottoman Turkish domination of the Mediterranean. In fact, records from the royal court reflect Pérez's repeated confirmation as royal surgeon appointed to the household of Don Juan until his patron's death.[33] Following the acclaimed victory of the Holy League at the Battle of Lepanto (1571), the Spanish fleet turned its attention to the recapture of Tunis from Ottoman control in 1573, which the Spaniards accomplished relatively easily. At this point, it appears that Daza Chacón made his way back to Spain, while Pérez remained with the garrison in Tunis, from which he was subsequently captured and then ransomed when Ottoman forces retook the city the next year.[34] Pérez later rejoined Don Juan's forces after the latter was appointed governor-general of the Netherlands in 1576 and remained there, even after Don Juan's death in 1578, until 1579 or 1580. Returning to Spain, Pérez was once again reunited with Andrés de León in the military forces amassed to take control of Portugal in 1580, an event that Daza Chacón narrowly missed, having been granted retirement by Philip only days before the expedition launched.[35] While Pérez and León headed to Portugal, Daza Chacón instead retired and worked on his voluminous surgical text, which also doubled as a sort of autobiography and memoir, the first part of which he published in 1582, with subsequent texts appearing in 1585 and 1595. The two remaining active surgeons, Pérez and León, both survived not only the relatively short Portuguese conquest, in which Spanish forces were successful after only one battle, but also the much more devastating failed Armada attack on England several years later in 1588.[36]

In addition to their active military travels and service, both Pérez and Léon wrote and published treatises on surgery (Pérez early in his career in 1568 and León much later in his in 1590), as well as later treatises on disease (Pérez on plague in 1598 and Léon on morbo gálico in 1605). The year 1605 marks the end of our knowledge of this contingent of learned military surgeons. Daza Chacón died sometime after 1596, the date at which he signed the approval for a license to publish for another learned surgeon, Bartolomé Hidalgo de Agüero. Antonio Pérez likely died in early 1605, as his widow petitioned the court for a pension in August of that year, recounting in it his long service to the crown.[37] Andrés de León published two treatises in 1605, one a compilation on surgery and anatomy in general and the other on morbo gálico. While it is likely he lived for some time after, no further records of him have been found.

Teaching and Practicing: Universities and Hospitals

Over half of the surgeons under consideration here were connected to royal patronage, either at court or in military service. The remaining four may be loosely categorized together as teachers of surgery. Only one of those is definitively known to have held a formal university position: Andrés Alcázar, who became the first professor of surgery at his alma mater, Salamanca. Two others, Juan Calvo in Valencia and Bartolomé Hidalgo de Agüero in Seville, were associated loosely with universities in those cities and taught surgery, though their connections to their respective universities are less clear. Juan Calvo attributed his decision to write (after twelve years of teaching) to his students who asked for an up-to-date manual of surgery. While the title page of his 1599 *Segunda parte de la medicina y cirugia* asserts his affiliation with the university as "Médico y lector de medicina en la Universidad de Valencia," he did not hold a *cátedra* or chair, but may have taught from his home.[38] Bartolomé Hidalgo de Agüero was head surgeon at one of Seville's hospitals, the Hospital del Cardinal, where he also taught students in surgery. While older biographers assumed he, too, held a chair at the university, this is unlikely, as the first chair of surgery there was created in 1592, only five years before his death. He certainly taught students, some of whom became dedicated followers of his practices, but within the hospital setting, not as a university master.[39] The fourth surgeon in the category of teachers, Francisco Arceo, likewise did some private teaching at his home, but mostly worked in various small towns between Badajoz and Seville. That these men were also important contributors to the surgical renaissance reflects the grassroots nature of this movement of change, pushed forward by many men who gained renown in their lifetimes despite having neither wealthy patrons nor prestigious positions but merely by practicing, teaching, and publishing texts.

Andrés Alcázar (c.1490–c. 1585) assumed the chair of surgery at the University of Salamanca upon its establishment in 1568. He was a product of that university, earning his doctor of medicine degree sometime in the first half of the century. He then spent a number of years practicing in Ávila, Segovia, and Guadalajara before assuming his position at the university where he remained until his death sometime around 1585.[40] Alcázar's text, *Chirurgiae libri sex* (1575) was a six-book work that devoted the first four books to wounds (head, nerves and tendons, chest, and abdomen) and the remaining two to disease (morbo gálico and bubonic plague). The first book, on head wounds, is considered Alcázar's greatest contribution to renaissance surgery and was reprinted as a stand-alone text in 1582.[41] In twenty-five chapters, Alcázar offers a thorough and detailed discussion of all types of head wounds, including their neurological symptoms and effects, as well as treatment methods.[42] In addition, Alcázar was a strong proponent of trepanation and developed a new form of trepan. His emphasis on neurology and innovations in instruments, in which he was joined by Francisco Arceo, are detailed further in the next chapter. Here it is sufficient to point out Alcázar's broader cultural influence as a professor at Salamanca, one of Spain's oldest and largest medical faculties, adding to both the geographic and career diversity of learned surgeons.

Joining Alcázar in his focus on head wounds was his contemporary Francisco Arceo (1493–1580), who shared other significant characteristics with Alcázar. Both men were born around the turn of the century, putting them into the older generation of learned surgeons, and both chose to write in Latin, contravening the wave of vernacular texts produced by their colleagues. Both composed only one major text, though Alcázar's first book was reprinted as a separate text, while Arceo's was translated into various vernaculars and therefore reprinted in various countries over the next century. Arceo's career and text stand out as unique in other ways as well. Though his knowledge of ancient authors is clear, Arceo's text is not an academic tome but is closer to the genre of *Observationes*, medical works written by physicians from the late sixteenth century onward, which compiled successful case studies.[43] He also offers various innovations in treatment, including the development of an orthopedic boot to correct clubfoot in children and the development of his own formula for a balsam or liniment to help wounds heal.[44] This Balsamo de Arceo became well-known, its recipe mentioned by other surgeons, including both Juan Fragoso and Bartolomé Hidalgo de Agüero, and continued to appear in pharmacological lists into the twentieth century.[45]

Arceo's educational training is unclear—older biographers state he was a graduate of Alcalá de Henares, but some more recent scholars have argued against this.[46] In either case, it is certain that he was well educated enough to know Latin and that he trained for some time in the hospitals of the Hieronymite monastery of Santa María de Guadalupe in Cáceres, which had become one of the best-known centers for medical (particularly surgical and anatomical) training in Castile. Arceo refers to a case he encountered while serving there in 1516 when he would have been twenty-three or twenty-four. Likely, then, he was continuing to hone his skills at Guadalupe before launching himself into a private career. Several other well-known physicians and surgeons likewise spent time working at Guadalupe, two of whom would become part of the intellectual circle of Seville to which Arceo also later became connected: Simón de Tovar, whose botanical garden of New World plants later brought him international recognition, and Francisco Hernández, who was also deeply interested in botanical materia medica and who we have already seen became friends with Juan Fragoso while both were in Seville.[47] Precisely how long Arceo remained in Guadalupe is unclear, but it does not seem to be more than a few years.

Francisco Arceo's career was one of both private and public practice, with occasional teaching. He spent his life just north of Seville, in the region of Badajoz, working in the towns of Fregenal de la Sierra, Fuente de Cantos, and Llerena, where he was employed at various times by both town authorities and the Inquisition.[48] Over the years, Arceo also taught a handful of students privately, including three who later went on to royal service.[49] His most famous student, Benito Arias Montano (1527–98), was neither physician nor surgeon, but a churchman and philosopher.

Francisco Arceo and Benito Arias Montano were both from Fregenal de la Sierra, a small town outside of Badajoz. An intellectual with close ties to Philip II's court, Arias Montano is another well-known figure to scholars of early modern Spain.[50] Among his many accomplishments, of most relevance here was the creation and maintenance of a network of scientific intellectuals that linked Seville and Antwerp. Arias Montano's deep interest in natural philosophy led him to what today would be considered the intersection of religion and science. Orphaned at an early age but well educated, Arias Montano undertook studies at both the University of

Seville and Alcalá de Henares. Later ordained a priest and a member of the Order of Santiago (St. James), he spent time in 1559 preaching in the town of Llerena, at the behest of his friend Francisco Arceo, with whom he stayed.[51] While there, he also undertook the study of surgery with Arceo, a reflection of both Arceo's reputation and Arias Montano's hunger for a wide range of knowledge, which he recounted in the preface he composed for Arceo's surgical text over a decade later. Arias Montano thereafter continued his rise to prominence in the church, attending part of the Council of Trent and then becoming a royal chaplain in 1566. Two years later, he was chosen by Philip II to oversee the publication of a new polyglot Bible at the printing press of Christophe Plantin in Antwerp.[52] Arias Montano spent the next seven years in this task, becoming enmeshed in the circle of scientists then actively publishing with Plantin, including cartographer Abraham Ortelius, mathematician Gemma Frisius, and botanist Carolus Clusius, as well as others.[53] He also acted as a book buyer, acquiring books and manuscripts on behalf of Philip II for the new library of the Escorial, as well as for friends back in Seville.[54]

While his contact with Plantin expanded Arias Montano's own intellectual circle, his lifelong ties to Seville helped forge a communication network that bridged Seville and Antwerp. Seville's prominence in the sixteenth century grew alongside its population, as it became the monopoly port for New World traffic and the center of the *Casa de la Contratación* (House of Trade) in 1503. The resultant growth of the city, in institutions, bureaucracy, infrastructure, and population meant that by the end of the century, it was the largest city in Spain and among the largest in Europe, with a population estimated around 100,000.[55] At the same time, the city also gained its own university, sanctioned by the crown in 1502 and the Papacy in 1505.[56] Yet while the university attracted scholars and trained many local intellectuals, it arguably was not what made Seville an intellectual center. Rather, the growing population and wealth in the city meant growing opportunities for patronage and the growth of various intellectual and cultural networks.[57] In addition, the economic opportunities of trade bolstered scientific inquiry, and Seville grew into an entrêpot that offered both economic and intellectual opportunities.[58] The city's printing presses produced more scientific volumes than any other city in Spain, publishing in both Latin and Castilian.[59] The intellectual and trade networks of Seville reached not only across Spain to Madrid and Valencia but also to the New World, Italy, and the Low Countries.[60]

During and after his years in Antwerp, Benito Arias Montano played a key role in connecting Seville's learned scientific and medical men with the work of colleagues across Europe. A dedicated bibliophile, Arias Montano acted as an agent for a variety of his friends in Spain, including Francisco Arceo and physicians Simón de Tovar and Nicolas Monardes. He acquired books on their behalf, oversaw the publication of Arceo's surgical text at Plantin's press in 1574, and fostered introductions and correspondence with the leading botanist of the time, Carolus Clusius (Charles L'Ecluse). Both Monardes and Tovar were practicing physicians with an interest in New World botany, and both maintained their own networks with family and friends in the Americas who sent or brought them seeds, cuttings, and plant samples, which they attempted to grow in private botanic gardens. As a result of these efforts, Monardes published several volumes describing New World materia medica, while Tovar corresponded with other botanists and began publishing a catalogue of his garden and available seeds or plants.[61] Clusius had traveled in Spain and Portugal in 1564–5, cataloguing plants and connecting with botanists, though there is no evidence that he met either Monardes or Tovar while stopping in Seville on that trip.[62] At some point, however, he received a copy of Monardes's text on New World materia medica and translated it into Latin, publishing it in two volumes with Plantin in 1574 and 1582. Clusius was also in correspondence with other naturalists in Seville, including Juan de Castañeda and Rodrigo Zamorano.[63] These men were one small part of Clusius's vast correspondence network stretching from the Low Countries to Denmark, Spain, Italy, and Austria.[64] Many medical intellectuals in Seville were thus interwoven into broader European exchanges of books, plants, seeds, and information.

Alongside the royal court in Madrid, the circle of medical intellectuals in Seville is one of the significant threads of connection among many of the learned surgeons under consideration here. Several men moved to join Philip II's court after working in Seville, including the previously mentioned Francisco Hernández and Juan Fragoso, as well as physician Andrés Zamudio de Alfaro who first served Philip II as *médico de camara* and later as Protomédico. The Seville circle also included many other well-known physicians, surgeons, and apothecaries. Prominent transplants to the city included the Valencian physician Francisco Franco, who settled in Seville as primary professor of medicine at the university after serving in similar positions at Alcalá de Henares and the University of Coimbra in Portugal, as well as serving as royal physician for King João III of Portugal; Miguel Martínez de Leyva, author of an early treatise on dentistry as well as one on plague; and Francisco Sánchez de Oropesa, a native of Toledo who was educated at Salamanca and who later also produced treatises on plague.[65] Other members of the Seville circle were natives to the city, including Zamudio de Alfaro, Nicolas Monardes, and Bartolomé Hidalgo de Agüero.

Bartolomé Hidalgo de Agüero was the only one of the surgeons under consideration here who did not ever leave the city of his birth. He studied at the University of Seville, learning surgery from Juan de la Cueva at the Hospital del Cardenal who he later replaced there as head surgeon.[66] Founded in 1455 by Cardenal Juan de Cervantes, the hospital's formal name was the Hospital de San Hermenegildo, but it was more commonly known as the Hospital del Cardenal or the Hospital de las heridas for the wounds it became specialized in treating. Hidalgo de Agüero did not initiate this specialization, but he certainly benefited from it, developing his own method of wound treatment, which he called the *vía particular*. In addition, Hidalgo de Agüero taught many students of his own at the hospital, several of whom went on to become authors themselves, including Juan de Sosa Sotomayor and Pedro López de Leon. Hidalgo de Agüero's work (and the debate it engendered) became so well-known that other Spanish surgeons who had not been his students also took up the question of his methods including Enrique Vaca de Alfaro and Pedro Gago de Vadilla.[67]

Hidalgo de Agüero's text was not traditional in structure, for he ignored the standard organization of information by body parts (generally head to toe) or types of conditions (such as wounds, ulcers, fractures, and so forth). Instead, he focused on advocating for his *vía particular*, sometimes referred to as the "dry" method, as opposed to the *vía común*, the standard or "wet" method.[68] In essence, Hidalgo de Agüero's new approach was a rejection of many of the interventions that were standard manipulation of wounds, such as enlarging wounds to better assess damage, the use of stents for drainage, cranial trepanation for head wounds, and other practices. Instead, he advocated for surgeons to intervene as little as possible, aside from keeping wounds clean and resetting fractures and breaks. The "dry" method refers to a rejection of the use of ointments or salves and heavy bandages for open wounds, which were standard by the sixteenth century. Several earlier medieval surgeons had advocated a similar approach, but it had fallen out of general favor. Hidalgo de Agüero may well have read some of these earlier texts, though he asserts throughout his writing that this was his own system, developed empirically in his work at the hospital and proven effective there as well. He certainly faced challenges to this new approach, as discussed in the next chapter, but he was very successful in his work at the Hospital del Cardenal and earned wide recognition for his skills. He seems to have had the support of the local city council, as well as of the circle of medical intellectuals in the city. His surgical text, *Thesoro de la verdadera cirugía y vía particular contra la común* (1604), published posthumously by his son-in-law, Francisco Jiménez Guillen, received royal approval for publication in 1596 from Dionisio Daza Chacón, who had retired from active royal service but was apparently still advising the crown.[69] His popular reputation outside of learned circles is reflected in the assertion made by biographers from the sixteenth century on that the young men in Seville often commended themselves to both God and to Hidalgo de Agüero before fights.[70] This phrase was first reported by Francisco Pacheco, a well-known artist (and father-in-law to court painter Diego Velázquez), who included Hidalgo de Agüero among the illustrious men whose sketch portraits and brief biographies he compiled in the *Libro de descripción de verdaderos retratos de ilustres y memorables varones* (1599; see Figure 2.1).[71]

The fourth teaching surgeon, Juan Calvo (1536–99), offers further geographic diversity as he lived and worked in Aragon rather than Castile. He earned his degrees in Valencia, studying under Luis Collado, a well-known anatomist who had studied with Vesalius and then continued further study in Zaragoza with another learned surgeon, Jerónimo Murillo.[72] After some years in Montpellier, France, he returned to Valencia in 1568, where he taught surgery. His study and subsequent work in Valencia placed him within another one of Iberia's principal centers of medical study and innovation. Valencia had been home to a school of surgery, *Estudi di Cirugía*, since the mid-fifteenth century and remained an influential center of medical studies through the following centuries.[73] The foundation of the university in 1499 incorporated the school of surgery, leading to the creation of chairs of medicine, surgery, and anatomy and simples by 1502. The last of these, a single position, combined wintertime dissections of corpses and springtime investigations of field botany. The two fields were later separated in 1560, adding to the number of medical chairs at the university. By the end of the century, the creation of

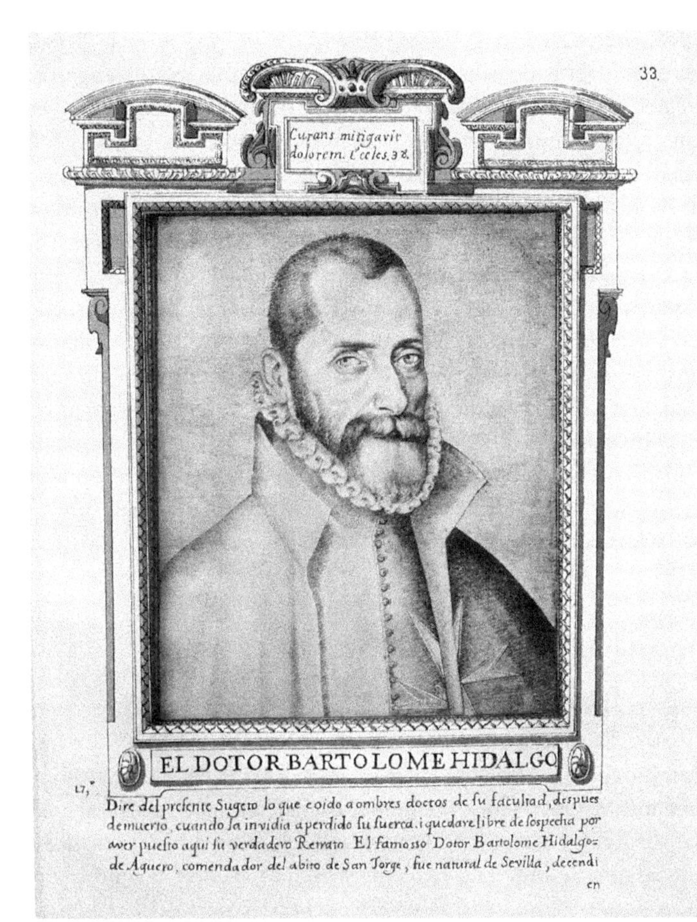
33.
Curans mitigavit dolorem. Eccles. 38.
EL DOTOR BARTOLOME HIDALGO
Dire del presente Sugeto lo que e oido a ombres doctos de su facultad, despues demuerto, cuando la invidia a perdido su suerca. i quedare libre de sospecha por aver puesto aqui su verdadero Retrato El famosso Dotor Bartolome Hidalgo de Aguero, comendador del abito de San Jorge, fue natural de Sevilla, decendi en

FIGURE 2.1 Portrait of Bartolomé Hidalgo de Agüero, from Francisco Pacheco, *Book of Portraits of Illustrious and Memorable Men* (1599).

additional chairs of practice meant the University of Valencia hosted a remarkable eight chairs of medicine, contrasted with the more common three or four at most other universities.[74] Among the men who held those chairs were several well-known medical humanists who helped keep Valencia on the intellectual cutting edge. In the first half of the sixteenth century, Miguel Jerónimo Ledesma (c. 1510–47), Pedro Jaime Esteve (c.1500–56), and Pedro Jimeno (c. 1515–51) studied abroad and then returned to Valencia to teach not only medicine, anatomy, and botany but also Greek, linguistics, and mathematics. Pedro Jimeno and Luis Collado introduced Vesalian anatomy to the city and the rest of the peninsula. Jimeno subsequently left Valencia for Alcalá de Henares, working alongside Francisco Valles. While Jimeno died soon thereafter, he influenced both Valles and Francisco Díaz, the learned royal surgeon.[75] Valencia also remained an influential center for medical studies and innovation.

Juan Calvo's text, *Primera y segunda parte de la cirugía universal* (1580), written for students after over a decade of teaching, covers the broad range of problems surgeons treated, including abscesses, wounds, fractures, dislocations, contusions, and abrasions. Calvo himself was not particularly innovative as a surgeon but may be seen instead as a compiler and translator of knowledge. A mark of his traditionalism is his 1596 publication of a new Castilian translation of Guy de Chauliac's 1363 text. Guy de Chauliac, referred to as simply Guido in Spanish texts, remained an important authority for learned surgeons. Chauliac's text was an authoritative model though, ironically, a work generally superseded by those of sixteenth-century learned surgeons. In fact, Calvo himself largely replaced Chauliac's text with his own enormously popular one, which was reprinted frequently through the next century, until 1703. On the other hand, Calvo can be seen as part of the surgical renaissance, as he was certainly well educated and embraced the use of the vernacular rather than Latin, enabling practitioners with varying education access to this knowledge. In addition, he kept abreast of the work of his more innovative contemporaries, whose works collectively account for roughly 40% of the references in his text.[76]

Print Networks

Learned surgeons, regardless of their location or type of practice, were embedded in the wider European medical Republic of Letters. A crucial component of learned texts, indeed the "learned" part of them, was their framing of information around other authoritative texts. References to ancient and medieval authors show Renaissance surgeons enmeshed in the intellectual world of textual knowledge, while references to contemporary texts (by which I mean those within the sixteenth century) show authors enmeshed in broader scholarly networks and embracing the intellectual shifts of their era. While we do not have correspondence collections for any of these Spanish surgeons, textual references provide a further way to understand their connections to each other as well as to other medical authors. These references show a circulation of knowledge and texts across national (and sometimes confessional) borders often otherwise unseen. That so many sixteenth-century medical scholars were so often cited by each other reflects the ongoing process by which new knowledge was being accumulated, tested, and legitimized in this era. The processes of legitimization and spread of knowledge are examined further in subsequent chapters. Here we will focus on the connections revealed among Spanish scholars and between Spanish and other European medical authors.

Citing Each Other

As shown at the outset of this chapter, a measure of the intellectual connections of these surgeons can be found in their citations of one another. Each author sought to add his own voice to the chorus of texts available in the late sixteenth century, deliberately choosing his own focus and organization. As learned practitioners, they clearly kept up with new publications of their colleagues, and they addressed each other's work, both positively and negatively. As a cohort publishing within the same generation, of course, surgeons could only cite work published before their own. A good example is Juan Fragoso, whose first text, *Erotemas chirurgicos* (1570), does not refer to any of his contemporary Spanish surgeons because this was one of the earliest publications by this cohort. He does include references to many other scholars from the earlier part of the sixteenth century, even providing at the outset a list of authors referred to.[77] Fragoso lists fifty-seven such authors, ranging from the expected ancients such as Hippocrates and Galen to the rather surprising Socrates and Homer. These two (and others) are referred to briefly in the dedicatory letter (to Diego de Espinosa, Bishop of Sigüenza, Inquisitor General, and president of the Council of Castile) and appear to be included in this list to show Fragoso's general erudition. Such references aside, there are over twenty authorities listed who worked in the first decades of the sixteenth century, including Giovanni da Vigo (1450–1525), Jean Fernel (1497–1558), and Andreas Vesalius (1514–64). Among these are numerous Spanish physicians, including Andrés Laguna (c.1510–59), Cristóbal de Vega (c.1510–c.1573), Francisco Valles (1524–92), Pedro Jaime Esteve (c. 1500–56), Luis Collado (c. 1520–89), and Juan Tomas Porcell (1528–c.1580).

A decade later, Fragoso rewrote and expanded his text, now titled *Cirugia universal* (1581). This later rendition no longer included the list of authors cited, but Fragoso continued to stay abreast of new publications, including in the updated edition numerous references to Francisco Arceo (published 1574), Andrés Alcázar (published 1575), and Juan Calvo (published 1580). That he read their texts closely is shown by his recounting of some of the particular cases given by them, as well as numerous general references to their work.[78]

For much of the text, Fragoso refers to his contemporary surgeons positively, though often indirectly. He does not mention them individually, often referring in the text to "alguno doctor," then citing (for example) Alcázar or Arceo in the marginal notes.[79] In his disagreements with others, he ranges from gently corrective to vehemently dismissive. In a discussion of facial wounds, Fragoso politely disagrees with contemporaries, stating, "Francisco Arceo and Giovanni da Vigo advise (though in different ways) to heal facial wounds with poultices, but in my opinion there is no better poultice than ordinary stitches made with a needle."[80] Fragoso's most dramatic disagreement was with Bartolomé Hidalgo de Agüero. Following Hidalgo de Agüero's first publication (a simple broadsheet of advice) in 1584, Fragoso appended an entire new treatise to the 1586 edition of his *Cirugia universal*, responding directly to (and negating much of the advice in) this broadsheet, a dispute addressed in detail in the next chapter.

Hidalgo de Agüero did not refer to any contemporaries in his initial 1584 broadsheet publication, but his subsequent text, completed in the 1590s, is replete with references. These include many sixteenth-century surgeons such as Berengario da Carpi, Amato Lusitano, and Vido Vidio, as well as his Spanish colleagues Arceo and Alcázar. His work is also notable, though, for his sustained response to Fragoso's attack on his earlier work, which is fifty folios long.[81] In addition, Hidalgo de

Agüero takes several smaller jabs at Fragoso. In the Antidotary, for example, he accuses Fragoso of misunderstanding Avicenna regarding the so-called Apostolic Unguent. According to Hidalgo de Agüero, Fragoso incorrectly cites Avicenna as attributing the name of this compound as coming from the fact that it was used by Christ's disciples. Hidalgo de Agüero shows us his close reading of both Fragoso and Avicenna by pointing out that Avicenna says no such thing, but rather says that it is called so because of its twelve ingredients, matching the number of disciples.[82] Hidalgo de Agüero also includes multiple references to both Arceo and Alcázar, though in more positive terms, for example repeating several recipes for ointments from Arceo.[83]

Hidalgo de Agüero was not the only surgeon to take issue with some of Fragoso's work. Juan Calvo also argued explicitly against Fragoso. For example, he begins the second part of his text by defining an ulcer as a "solution of continuity of the flesh in which there are certain aspects which impede the reunification and cure. This is a good fundamental definition and describes well the nature of an ulcer; although Fragoso says differently in his commentary."[84] Calvo not only disputes Fragoso on his definitions but also takes him to task directly on many other points. José Luis Fresquet Febrer's study of Calvo's text argues that just over 5% of all references Calvo makes are to Fragoso. Indeed, Fragoso's name is scattered throughout the text, appearing in passages across all topics. The posthumous 1626 edition of Calvo's text includes a listing of "errores de Fragoso" at the end of the alphabetical index, though this lists only six specific ideas. As noted earlier, Calvo also refers to numerous modern authors, including Berendagio da Carpi, Realdo Colombo, Gabriel Falloppio, and Andreas Vesalius, as well as his Spanish contemporaries Andrés Alcázar and Dionisio Daza Chacón.[85]

Referencing Others

All the surgeons under consideration here refer nearly constantly to ancient medical authorities, frequently to medieval ones, and periodically to modern or contemporary ones. Some, like Fragoso, include at the beginning of their texts a list of authors referred to, both ancient and modern. Fragoso's previously mentioned fifty-seven authors become paltry in comparison to Francisco Díaz's *Compendio*, which lists eighty-seven, and Daza Chacón's *Practica y teorica*, which includes an alphabetical listing of a whopping 214 authors. These reference lists are not necessarily inclusive of all such references, but we can understand them as a kind of signaling to readers of the author's erudition. Dionisio Daza Chacón's massive list of authors has far more ancient authorities than contemporaries, not only medical but also literary and philosophical. Thus, in addition to the universal figures of Hippocrates, Galen, and Celsus, we find other ancient medical authors such as Caelius Aurelianus, Alexander of Tralles, and Philoxenus alongside figures as varied as Seneca, Aristophanes, and Diodorus Siculus. Alongside medieval medical figures such as Lanfranc, Guy de Chauliac (Guido), and Bernard of Gordon (Gordonio) are humanists Poggio Bracciolini (Pogio Florentino), Giovanni Boccaccio, and George of Trebizond (Georgio Trapeçuncio). Daza Chacón was unusual in his heavy balance of ancient authorities, with scarce references to his sixteenth-century contemporaries. Among sixteenth-century authors he referenced were Andrés Laguna and Francisco Valles, along with Giovanni da Vigo, Bartolomeo Eustachi (Eustachio, 15014?–74), and Amato Lusitano (João Rodrigues de Castelo Branco, 1511–68).

Amato Lusitano's work is referred to in most Spanish learned surgical texts, despite suffering censorship by the Spanish Inquisition.[86] He was a Portuguese Jewish physician who studied medicine at Salamanca. He then spent his career in exile, moving first to Antwerp and then to Ferrara, Ancona, Ragusa, and Thessaloniki, partly in order to avoid persecution. His most famous work, composed over the course of a decade (1551–61), comprised seven volumes of a hundred case studies each. The work was placed on numerous Indices of prohibited books in Portugal, Spain, and Rome from 1581 onward.[87] Expurgated editions, in which offending passages were removed, were permitted by all three Inquisitions, however, so it is not entirely surprising to find his work referenced by so many. In fact, the late date of appearance in the Indices (twenty years after the final volume appeared in print) means that many, like Francisco Díaz, wrote before the earliest condemnations appeared. Lusitano was not the only medical authority who appeared on the Spanish Index of Forbidden Books, though he was the one most commonly cited. Among others, we find Arnaldo de Villanova (Arnau de Vilanova), Leonardo Fioravanti, and Conrad Gesner.[88] Not all the works of each of these authors were on the index, and those that were simply needed to be expurgated. In his treatise in response to Hidalgo de Agüero, Juan Fragoso quotes Conrad Gesner's criticism of Paracelsus, carefully noting after that his copy of Paracelsus's *Cirurgia magna* is properly expurgated.[89] These citations are an additional reminder of how widely medical texts circulated, even across confessional lines, and how well-read learned surgeons were.

By far the contemporary learned surgeon most often cited by Spaniards was Giovanni da Vigo, the papal surgeon whose 1516 *Practica in arte chirurgica copiosa* received numerous translations and reprinting, becoming a standard across much of Europe. Other notable surgeon-anatomists commonly cited included Berengario da Carpi, Gabrielle Falloppio, and Guido Guidi (Vido Vidio, 1508?–69), a Florentine surgeon and anatomist who served as royal physician to Francis I of France and Cosimo de Medici, as well as a professor at the University of Pisa.[90] The Italian botanist Pietro Andrea Mattioli (1501–77) was cited by several Spaniards, including Fragoso, Díaz, and Arceo. Finally, the well-known French surgeon Ambroise Paré, an important innovator and prolific author, appears at least once in nearly all the Spanish texts studied here.

Learned surgeons formed an intellectual community connected together personally and professionally in overlapping circles of education, geography, specialization, experience, and career path. They were also linked to medical practitioners throughout Europe and the Americas who were similarly utilizing their knowledge and skills to promote surgery as a learned profession, grounded in ancient authority and explicated in printed texts. Working in a broad range of contexts (at court, as private practitioners, in military service), these men were both practitioners and educators who developed innovative techniques, consolidated knowledge, and demonstrated the importance of university education for surgeons. Knowledgeable in traditional texts, these surgeons were then able to balance ancient theories against modern experience, embracing the new technology of printing to promote their ideas and disperse their knowledge.

Notes

1 Juan Calvo, *Primera y segunda parte de la Cirugia uniuersal y particular del cuerpo humano* (Madrid: Diego Flamenco, 1626), 288.
2 Juan Fragoso, *Cirugia universal … Y mas otros tres tratados … El primero es, una summa de proposiciones contraciertos avisos de cirugia. El segundo, de las declaraciones acerca de diversas heridas y muertos. El tercero, de los Aphorismos de Hyppocrates tocantes a cirugia*, 1592, fols. 143v–44.
3 Florike Egmond, *The World of Carolus Clusius: Natural History in the Making, 1550–1610*, Perspectives in Economic and Social History, no. 6 (Brookfield, Vt: Pickering & Chatto, 2010); Josep Lluís Barona and Xavier Gómez Font, *La correspondencia de Carolus Clusius con los científicos españoles* (València: Universitat de València, 1998); Peter N. Miller, *Peiresc's Mediterranean World* (Cambridge, MA: Harvard University Press, 2017); A. Rupert Hall, Marie Boas, *The Correspondence of Henry Oldenburg*, 9 vols. (Madison, WI: University of Wisconsin Press, 1965).
4 Mordechai Feingold, ed., *Jesuit Science and the Republic of Letters*, Transformations (Cambridge, MA: MIT Press, 2003); A. Lynn Martin, *Plague?: Jesuit Accounts of Epidemic Disease in the 16th Century* (Kirksville, MO: Sixteenth Century Journal Publishers, 1996).
5 Paula Findlen, *Possessing Nature: Museums, Collecting, and Scientific Culture in Early Modern Italy*, Studies on the History of Society and Culture 20 (Berkeley: University of California Press, 1994); Ole Peter Grell, Andrew Cunningham, and Jon Arrizabalaga, eds., *Centres of Medical Excellence? Medical Travel and Education in Europe 1500–1789* (Burlington, VT: Ashgate, 2010); Luis García Ballester, Jon Arrizabalaga, and Fernando Salmón, "A propósito de las relaciones intelectuales entre la Corona de Aragón e Italia (1470–1520): Los estudiantes de medicina valencianos en los estudios generales de Siena, Pisa, Ferrara y Padua," *Dynamis: Acta Hispanica ad Medicinae Scientiarumque Historiam Illustrandam* 9 (1989): 117–47; Timothy Walker, "Aquisition and Circulation of Medical Knowledge within the Early Modern Portuguese Colonial Empire," in *Science in the Spanish and Portuguese Empires, 1500–1800*, ed. Daniela Bleichmar et al. (Stanford, CA: Stanford University Press, 2009); Nancy G. Siraisi, *Communities of Learned Experience: Epistolary Medicine in the Renaissance* (Baltimore, MD: Johns Hopkins University Press, 2013).
6 See, for example, Luis S. Granjel, *Cirugía Española Del Renacimiento* (Salamanca: Universidad de Salamanca, 1968); José Luis Fresquet Febrer, "La práctica médica en los textos quirúrgicos españoles en el siglo XVIII," *Dynamis: Acta Hispanica Ad Medicinae Scientiarumque Historiam Illustrandam* 22 (2002): 251–77; Ana I. Martín Ferreira, "El ideal de Celso en la cirugía española del s. XVI," *Medizinhistorisches Journal* 30, no. 2 (1995): 145–65; José María López Piñero, *Ciencia y técnica en la sociedad española de los siglos XVI y XVII* (Barcelona: Labor Universitaria, 1979), 361–8.
7 López Piñero, *Ciencia y técnica en la sociedad española de los siglos XVI y XVII*, 361–8.
8 Juan Fragoso, *Catalogus simplicium medicamentorum* (Alcalá de Henares: P. Robles & J. Villanoua, 1566); Juan Fragoso, *Discurso de las cosas aromaticas, arboles y frutales y de otras muchas medicinas simples que se traen de la India Oriental y que siruen al vso de medicina* (Madrid: en casa de Francisco Sanchez, 1572); Juan Fragoso, *De succedaneis medicamentis liber denuo auctus … Ejusdem animadversiones, in quamplurima medicamenta composita, quoru[m] est usus in hispanicis officinis* (Madrid, 1575).

9 Geoffrey Parker, *Imprudent King: A New Life of Philip II* (New Haven, CT: Yale University Press, 2014), 100–1.
10 William Eamon, "The Charlatan's Trial. An Italian Surgeon in the Court of King Phillip II, 1576–1577," *Cronos. Cuadernos Valencianos de Historia de La Medicina y de La Ciencia* 8 (2000): 4; David C. Goodman, *Power and Penury: Government, Technology, and Science in Philip II's Spain* (New York: Cambridge University Press, 1988), 230–33; Michele L Clouse, *Medicine, Government and Public Health in Philip II's Spain: Shared Interests, Competing Authorities* (Burlington, VT: Ashgate, 2011), 75–110.
11 Henry Kamen, *Philip of Spain* (New Haven, CT: Yale University Press, 1997), 208–9; Sagrario Muñoz Calvo, "El medicamento en la Medicina de Cámara de Felipe II: Protagonismo de Juan Fragoso," in *La Ciencia En El Monasterio Del Escorial*, ed. Francisco Javier Campos (Madrid: Ediciones Escurialenses, 1992), 246.
12 Parker, *Imprudent King*, 156–74.
13 Parker, 284.
14 Goodman, *Power and Penury*, 230; See also María Teresa Oliveros de Castro and Eliseo Subiza Martin, *Felipe II: Estudio Médico-Histórico*, Publicaciones de La Universidad de Madrid: Monografías Científicas (Madrid: Aguilar, 1956).
15 See, for example, the titles and salaries listed in Juan Manuel Jiménez Muñoz, *Médicos y cirujanos en "Quitaciones de Corte" (1435–1715)* (Valladolid: Universidad de Valladolid, 1977).
16 Luis S. Granjel, *La Medicina Española Renacentista*, Historia General de La Medicina Española, II (Salamanca: Universidad de Salamanca, 1980), 30–8.
17 Clouse, *Medicine, Government and Public Health in Philip II's Spain*, 75–6.
18 Eamon, "The Charlatan's Trial. An Italian Surgeon in the Court of King Phillip II, 1576–1577"; Clouse, *Medicine, Government and Public Health in Philip II's Spain*, 77–84; Francisco Díaz, *Tratado, nuevamente impresso, de todas las enfermedades de los riñones, vexiga, y carnosidades de la verga y urina: dividido en tres libros* (Madrid, 1588), 317–22; Gustav Ungerer, "George Baker: Translator of Aparicio de Zubia's Pamphlet on the 'Oleum Magistrale,'" *Medical History* 30, no. 02 (1986): 203–11, https://doi.org/10.1017/S0025727300045397.
19 Simon Varey, Rafael Chabrán, and Dora B. Weiner, eds., *Searching for the Secrets of Nature: The Life and Works of Dr. Francisco Hernández* (Stanford, CA: Stanford University Press, 2000); Francisco Hernández and Simon Varey, *The Mexican Treasury: The Writings of Dr. Francisco Hernández* (Stanford, CA: Stanford University Press, 2000).
20 M J Rodríguez Salgado, "«Una perfecta princesa». Casa y vida de la reina Isabel de Valois (1559–1568). Primera parte," *Cuadernos de Historia Moderna*, 2003, 89.
21 Alexander Samuel Wilkinson and Alejandra Ulla Lorenzo, eds., *Iberian Books Volumes II & III/Libros Ibéricos Volúmenes II y III (2 vols): Books Published in Spain, Portugal and the New World or Elsewhere in Spanish or Portuguese between 1601 and 1650/Libros publicados en España, Portugal y el Nuevo Mundo o Impresos en Otros Lugares en Español o Portugués entre 1601 y 1650* (Boston: Brill, 2015), 359.
22 Alexander S. Wilkinson, ed., *Iberian Books/Libros Ibéricos (IB): Books Published in Spanish or Portuguese or on the Iberian Peninsula before 1601/Libros publicados en español o portugués o en la Península Ibérica antes de 1601* (Boston: Brill, 2010), 359. See also the Universal Short Title Catalogue (www.ustc.ac.uk) and the National Library of Medicine's LocatorPlus catalogue (nlm.nih.gov).
23 Carlos Alberto González Sánchez, Tristán Platt, and Bethany Aram, *New World Literacy: Writing and Culture Across the Atlantic,1500–1700*, The Bucknell Studies in Latin American Literature and Theory (Lewisburg, PA: Bucknell University Press, 2011), 85, 119, 177, 224; Jose Torre Revello, *El Libro, La Imprenta y El Periodismo En América Durante La Dominación Española*, no. 74 (Buenos Aires: Publicaciones del Instituto de Investigaciones Historicas, 1940), 242; Linda A. Newson and Susie Minchin, *From Capture to Sale: The Portuguese Slave Trade to Spanish South America in the Early Seventeenth Century*, The Atlantic World, v. 12 (Leiden; Boston: Brill, 2007), 267–9.

24 Newson and Minchin, *From Capture to Sale*, 268; Carlos Alberto González Sánchez, *New World Literacy: Writing and Culture Across the Atlantic, 1500–1700*, trans. Tristán Platt and Bethany Aram (Lewisburg, PA: Bucknell University Press, 2011), 177.
25 José Antonio Perálvarez, "Francisco Díaz, Padre de La Urología," *Historias de Alcalá* (blog), Publicado el agosto 2015, https://historiasdealcala.wordpress.com/2015/08/03/francisco-diaz-padre-de-la-urologia/.
26 Perálvarez; Emilio Maganto Pavón, "Francisco Díaz," Historia de la Urología Española, n.d., http://historia.aeu.es/FranciscoDiaz.htm.
27 Juan Fragoso and Francisco Díaz, *Cirugia uniuersal, aora nueuamenta añadida...: Iten otros quatro tratados, el primero es una suma de proposiciones contra auisos de cirugia, el segundo de las declaraciones acerca de diuersas heridas y muertes, el tercero, de los Aphorismos de Hipocrates tocantes a cirugia, el cuarto, de la naturaleza y calidades de los medicamentos simples; Iten un tratado de todas las enfermedades de los riñones, vexiga y carnosidades de la verga y orina y de su cura...; por Francisco Diaz...* (por la viuda de Alonso Martin, 1627).
28 These cases are discussed further in Chapter 3. Daza Chacon's account of Henry II's head wound can be found in Dionisio Daza Chacón, *Practica y teorica de cirugia en romance y en latin* (Valladolid: en casa de Ana Velez, 1609), 205–6; See also Charles Donald O'Malley and J. B. de C. M. Saunders, "The 'Relation' of Andreas Vesalius on the Death of Henry II of France," *Journal of the History of Medicine and Allied Sciences* 3 (1948): 197–213; His account of Don Carlos' wound is found in Martín Fernández de Navarrete et al., eds., *Colección de Documentos Inéditos Para La Historia de España* (Madrid, 1842), 18: 537–63; and further analyzed in L. J. Andrew Villalon, "Putting Don Carlos Together Again: Treatment of a Head Injury in Sixteenth- Century Spain," *Sixteenth Century Journal* 26, no. 2 (1995): 347–65.
29 Andrés de León, *Practico de morbo gallico, en el qual se contiene el origen y conocimiento della enfermedad, y el mejor modo de curarla* (Valladolid, 1605), fol. 5v.
30 Nicolas Monardes, *Dos libros. El uno trata de todas las cosas que traen de nuestras Indias Occidentales, que siruen al uso de medicina, ... El otro libro, trata de los medicinas marauillosas que son contra todo veneno, la piedra Bezaar, y la yerua escuerçonera. Con la cura de los venenados. ... Agora nueuamente copuestos por el doctor Niculoso de Monardes medico de Seuilla* (Sevilla, 1565).
31 León, *Practico de morbo gallico*, fols. 5v–6.
32 Henry Kamen, *Spain, 1469–1714: A Society of Conflict*, Fourth edition (New York: Routledge, 2014), 130–2; 149–52.
33 Jiménez Muñoz, *Médicos y cirujanos en "Quitaciones de Corte" (1435–1715)*, 81.
34 Cristóbal Pérez Pastor, *Bibliografía madrileña o descripción de las obras impresas en Madrid* (Tipografía de los Huérfanos, 1907), 447.
35 Daza Chacón, *Practica y teorica*, prologo.
36 Pastor, *Bibliografía madrileña o descripción de las obras impresas en Madrid*, 447; León, *Practico de morbo gallico*, fols. 5v–6.
37 Pastor, *Bibliografía madrileña o descripción de las obras impresas en Madrid*, 447–8.
38 Jose Luis Fresquet Febrer, ed., *Juan Calvo y la cirugía valenciana del siglo XVI: Simposio 2002 sobre la historia de la medicina* (València: Editorial Denes, 2002), 63; José López Piñero et al., *Diccionario Histórico de La Ciencia Moderna En España*, 1a ed., vol. I (A–L) (Barcelona: Península, 1983), 160–1.
39 José Antonio Ollero Pina, *La Universidad de Sevilla en los siglos XVI y XVII* (Sevilla: Publicaciones de la Universidad de Sevilla, 1993), 413–14.
40 López Piñero et al., *Diccionario Histórico de La Ciencia Moderna En España*, I (A–L): 34–6.
41 Wilkinson, *Iberian Books/Libros Ibéricos (IB)*, 10; López Piñero et al., *Diccionario Histórico de La Ciencia Moderna En España*, I (A–L): 34.
42 Granjel, *Cirugía Española Del Renacimiento*, 67–9; Antonio Herrera Casado, "Andrés Alcázar, Cirujano Del Renacimiento," in *Gran Enciclopedia de Castilla-La Mancha*, vol. I (Zaragoza: Unión Aragonesa del Libro, 1982), 15; Luis S. Granjel, "La Obra de Andrés Alcázar," *Clínica Y Laboratorio* LXVII, no. 395 (1959): 154–60.

43 Gianna Pomata, "Sharing Cases: The *Observationes* in Early Modern Medicine," *Early Science and Medicine* 15, no. 3 (2010): 193–236, https://doi.org/10.1163/157338210X493932; Gianna Pomata, "Observation Rising: Birth of an Epistemic Genre, 1500–1650," in *Histories of Scientific Observation*, ed. Lorraine Daston and Elizabeth Lunbeck (Chicago, IL: University of Chicago Press, 2011), 45–80.

44 José Ramón Vallejo, Marina Mesa, and José M. Cobos-Bueno, "Francisco Arceo de Fregenal and the Treatment of Clubfoot up to the Sixteenth Century," *Acta Medico-Historica Adriatica* 16, no. 1 (2018): 19–48, https://doi.org/10.31952/amha.16.1.1; José M. Cobos-Bueno, Andrés Oyola Fabián, and Juan Fernando García Ávila, "El bálsamo de Francisco Arceo de Fregenal," *Llull* 33 (2010): 241–68.

45 Bartolomé Hidalgo de Agüero, *Thesoro de la verdadera cirugía y vía particular contra la común* (Sevilla: Francisco Pérez, 1604), fols. 113, 115v; Fragoso and Díaz, *Cirugia uniuersal, aora nueuamenta añadida…*, fol. 224v.

46 Francisco Arceo de Fregenal, *Método verdadero de curar las heridas y otros preceptos de este arte: Método de curar las fiebres*, ed. Andrés Oyola Fabián and J. Cobos Bueno, Bibliotheca Montaniana 21 (Huelva: Universidad de Huelva, 2009), 37–9; Enrique Montero Cartelle, "Benito Arias Montano y Francisco Arceo: la Redacción del De recta curandorum vulnerum ratione," *Asclepio* 64, no. 2 (2012): 418, https://doi.org/10.3989/asclepio.2012.v64.i2.527.

47 Sebastián García, "Medicina y Cirugía En Los Reales Hospitales de Guadalupe," *Revista de Estudios Extremeños* 59, no. 1 (2003): 67–9.

48 José Miguel Cobos and José Ramón Vallejo, "Francisco Arceo, médico del Santo Oficio de la Inquisición de Llerena," *Inquisición: XV Jornadas de historia en Llerena*, 2014, 299–310.

49 Cobos and Vallejo, 301.

50 A 2005 bibliography of studies about Arias Montano (since 1832) is over 35 pages long: Rafael Caso Amador, "Bibliografía Sobre El Humanista Benito Arias Montano (1832–2005)," *Etiópicas: Revista de Letras Renacentistas* 1 (2004–5): 271–304.

51 Ben Rekers, *Benito Arias Montano (1527–1598)*, Studies of the Warburg Institute 33 (Leiden: E.J. Brill, 1972), 3; María M. Portuondo, *The Spanish Disquiet: The Biblical Natural Philosophy of Benito Arias Montano* (Chicago: The University of Chicago Press, 2019), 22–4.

52 Portuondo, *The Spanish Disquiet*, 27.

53 "The Correspondence of Christophe Plantin," Early Modern Letters Online, accessed June 19, 2021, http://emlo-portal.bodleian.ox.ac.uk/collections/?catalogue=christophe-plantin; Portuondo, *The Spanish Disquiet*, 157–60; Rekers, *Benito Arias Montano (1527–1598)*, 74–5; López Piñero, *Ciencia y técnica en la sociedad española de los siglos XVI y XVII*, 144.

54 María M. Portuondo, "The Study of Nature, Philosophy, and the Royal Library of San Lorenzo of the Escorial," *Renaissance Quarterly* 63, no. 4 (2010): 1109–11, https://doi.org/10.1086/658508; Portuondo, *The Spanish Disquiet*, 157–79.

55 Antonio Domínguez Ortiz, *The Golden Age of Spain, 1516–1659*, trans. James Casey (New York: Basic Books, 1971).

56 Ollero Pina, *La Universidad de Sevilla en los siglos XVI y XVII*, 37–40. The university is often seen as an outgrowth of medieval schools of Latin and Arabic established in the city by King Alfonso X in 1254.

57 Guy Lazure, "To Dare Fame: Constructing a Cultural Elite in Sixteenth Century Seville" (Ph.D., Baltimore, MD, Johns Hopkins University, 2003).

58 Harold J. Cook, *Matters of Exchange: Commerce, Medicine, and Science in the Dutch Golden Age* (New Haven, CT: Yale University Press, 2007); Pamela H. Smith and Paula Findlen, eds., *Merchants and Marvels: Commerce, Science, and Art in Early Modern Europe* (New York: Routledge, 2002); Paula De Vos, "The Science of Spices: Empiricism and Economic Botany in the Early Spanish Empire," *Journal of World History* 17, no. 4 (2006): 399–427, https://doi.org/10.1353/jwh.2006.0054.

59 López Piñero, *Ciencia y técnica en la eociedad española de los siglos XVI y XVII*, 58–66.

60 Alonso Morgado, *Historia de Sevilla* (Sevilla, 1587); Lazure, "To Dare Fame: Constructing a Cultural Elite in Sixteenth Century Seville"; Kristy Wilson Bowers, "Tradition and Innovation in Spanish Medicine: Bartolomé Hidalgo de Agüero and the Vía Particular," *Sixteenth Century Journal* XLI, no. I (2010): 29–47; Carolina Abadia Flores, "La Comunidad Flamenca en Sevilla en el siglo XVI," *Archivo Hispalense: Revista Histórica, Literaria y Artística* 282–4 (2010): 173–92.

61 Miguel López Pérez and Mar Rey Bueno, "Simón de Tovar (1528–1596): redes familiares, naturaleza americana y comercio de maravillas en la Sevilla del XVI," *Dynamis: Acta Hispanica ad Medicinae Scientiarumque Historiam Illustrandam* 26, no. 0 (2006): 69–91; José Luis Fresquet Febrer, "La fundación y desarrollo de los jardines botánicos," in *Felipe II, la Ciencia y la Técnica*, ed. Enrique Martínez Ruiz (Madrid: Editorial Actas, 1999), 189.

62 Boxer, *Two Pioneers of Tropical Medicine*, 26; María Luz López Terrada, "Flora and the Hapsburg Crown: Clusius, Spain, and American Natural History," in *Silent Messengers: The Circulation of Material Objects of Knowledge in the Early Modern Low Countries*, ed. Sven Dupré and Christoph Lüthy (Berlin: LIT, 2011), 49.

63 López Terrada, "Flora and the Hapsburg Crown," 55.

64 Florike Egmond, *The World of Carolus Clusius: Natural History in the Making, 1550–1610*, (New York: Routledge, 2010); Florike Egmond et al., eds., *Carolus Clusius: Towards a Cultural History of a Renaissance Naturalist* (Amsterdam: Koninklijke Nederlandse Akademie van Wetenschappen, 2007).

65 Antonio Hernández Morejón, *Historia Bibliográfica de la Medicina Española (1842–1852)*, vol. III, 145–8, 382–6, 416–18. http://147.156.5.138/Morejon_Chinchilla/

66 Joaquín Herrera Dávila, *El Hospital del Cardenal de Sevilla y el Doctor Hidalgo de Agüero* (Sevilla: Fundación de Cultura Andaluza, 2010).

67 Bowers, "Tradition and Innovation in Spanish Medicine: Bartolomé Hidalgo de Agüero and the Vía Particular," 45–6.

68 The question of whether (or which) wounds should be treated with oils or drying agents was an old one, traceable in Hippocratic writings and revived in the Middle Ages. Nancy G. Siraisi, *Medieval & Early Renaissance Medicine: An Introduction to Knowledge and Practice* (Chicago: University of Chicago Press, 1990), 169–70; Leo M. Zimmerman and Ilza Veith, *Great Ideas in the History of Surgery*, 2d rev. ed (New York: Dover Publications, 1967), 16.

69 Charles Donald O'Malley, "Dionisio Daza Chacon," in *Medizingeschichte in Unserer Zeit. Festgabe Fur Edith Heischkel-Artelt Und Walter Artelt Zum 65. Geburtstag.*, ed. Hans-Heinz Eulner et al. (Stuttgart: Ferndinand Enke Verlag, 1971), 170.

70 This is reported variously as "Á Dios me encomiendo, y al doctor Hidalgo de Agüero" or "En Dios me encomiendo y en manos de Agüero." Pacheco (1599) seems to have been the initial source for this, and it has been repeated many times over by most biographers. Whether objectively true or not, Pacheco's inclusion of Hidalgo de Agüero in his work reflects his contemporary reputation in the city. See Chinchilla, II, p. 28; Morejón, III, p. 322; Pacheco, 154.

71 Marta Cacho Casal, "The 'True Likenesses' in Francisco Pacheco's Libro de Retratos: Francisco Pacheco's Libro de Retratos," *Renaissance Studies* 24, no. 3 (2010): 381–406, https://doi.org/10.1111/j.1477-4658.2009.00599.x.

72 Fresquet Febrer, *Juan Calvo y la cirugía valenciana del siglo XVI: Simposio 2002 sobre la historia de la medicina*, 63; López Piñero et al., *Diccionario Histórico de La Ciencia Moderna En España*, I (A-L): 234–6.

73 Mercedes Gallent Marco, "El Colegio de Barberos y Cirujanos de Valencia: Aportación Documental," *Saitabi: revista de la Facultat de Geografia i Història* 43 (1993): 147–56; Bjørn Okholm Skaarup, *Anatomy and Anatomists in Early Modern Spain* (Burlington, VT: Ashgate, 2015), 33–63.

74 Luis García Ballester, "La cirugía en la Valencia del siglo XV. El privilegio de desecar cadaveres en 1477," *Cuadernos de Historia de La Medicina Espanola* 7 (1967): 158; José M. López Piñero, "The Faculty of Medicine of Valencia," in *Universities and Science in the Early Modern Period*, ed. Mordechai Feingold and Víctor Navarro Brotons, Archimedes, v. 12 (Dordrecht: Springer, 2006), 68.

75 Díaz, *Tratado, nuevamente impresso, de todas las enfermedades de los riñones, vexiga, y carnosidades de la verga y urina*, 19–19v.
76 Fresquet Febrer, *Juan Calvo y la cirugía valenciana del siglo XVI: Simposio 2002 sobre la historia de la medicina*, 67.
77 Juan Fragoso, *Erotemas chirurgicos en los que se enseña todo lo mas necessario del arte de cyrurgia…* (por Pierres Cosin, a costa de Sebastian Yuañez, 1570), n.p. "Los autores de quien este libro se hace mencion."
78 For particular case studies, see Fragoso, *Cirugia universal*, fols. 92, 143v–4 and passing references, for example, on ff. 56, 59v, 271v.
79 Fragoso, fols. 55v, 56, 59v.
80 "Francisco Arceo, y Juan de Vigo enseñan (aunque a diferentes maneras) a curar heridas del rostro con cataplasmas, aunque a mi parecer no ay mejor cataplasma que la costura ordinaria bien hecha con el aguja." Fragoso, fol. 146v.
81 "Respuesta del dotor Hidalgo a el Licenciado Fragoso," Bartolomé Hidalgo de Agüero, *Thesoro de la verdadera cirugía y vía particular contra la común* (Sevilla: Francisco Pérez, 1604), fols. 144–93.
82 Bartolomé Hidalgo de Agüero, *Thesoro de la verdadera cirugía y vía particular contra la común* (Sevilla: Francisco Pérez, 1604), fol. 114.
83 Bartolomé Hidalgo de Agüero, *Thesoro de la verdadera cirugía y vía particular contra la común* (Sevilla: Francisco Pérez, 1604), fols. 113–15v.
84 "[S]olucion en continuidad en la carne en la qual se hallan ciertas disposiciones, que impiden la union, y curacion. Esta diffinicion es buena y essencial, y verdaderamente declara la naturaleza y essencia de la ulcera; aunque diga Fragoso en su glossa lo contrario." Juan Calvo, *Segunda parte de la medicina y cirurgia, que trata de las vlceras en general y particular, y del Antidotario, en el qual se trata de la facultad de todos los medicame[n]tos assi simples como compuestos segun Gal. en el libro quarto y quinto de la facultad de los simples, con otros tratados* (Valencia, 1599), 2.
85 Fresquet Febrer, *Juan Calvo y la cirugía valenciana del siglo XVI: Simposio 2002 sobre la historia de la medicina*, 66–7.
86 Isilda Rodrigues and Carlos Fiolhais, "La censura inquisitorial en las Centurias de Amatus Lusitanus," *Asclepio: Revista de Historia de La Medicina y de La Ciencia* 70, no. 2 (December 20, 2018): 229, https://doi.org/10.3989/asclepio.2018.13; Dov Front, "The Expurgation of Medical Books in Sixteenth-Century Spain," *Bulletin of the History of Medicine* 75, no. 2 (2001): 290–6, https://doi.org/10.1353/bhm.2001.0067.
87 Front, "The Expurgation of Medical Books in Sixteenth-Century Spain," 291.
88 José Pardo Tomás, "Autores médicos en los índices inquisitoriales españoles del siglo XVI," *Dynamis: Acta Hispanica Ad Medicinae Scientiarumque Historiam Illustrandam; Vol. 5–6* 5 (January 1, 1985).
89 Fragoso and Díaz, *Cirugia uniuersal, aora nueuamenta añadida…*, fol. 514 "tuve en mi poder la Cirugia Magna y Parva del dicho Teofrastro Paracelso, expurgada conforme al nuevo catalogo, y expurgatorio del santo oficio, por el Doctor Juan de Llano, impressa Argentorati, anno 1573."
90 William Brockbank, "The Man Who Was Vidius," *Annals of The Royal College of Surgeons of England* 19, no. 5 (1956): 269–95.

3

SHARING KNOWLEDGE

Learned Surgical Texts

Dionisio Daza Chacón begins his text with an address to the reader: "Before giving account of my work and travels (gentle reader) I would like to recount my motivation for writing in Spanish, rather than in Latin, which would certainly have been much easier and less work for me: the reason is evident because if I wrote in Latin, it would not be necessary to look for the proper interpretation of words that surgeons use, nor to translate the texts of ancient and modern writers, which has caused me great work, but I would render in Latin what they wrote in Latin."[1] He goes on to state that he found it both necessary and useful to go to the trouble of writing in the vernacular because after having worked for twelve years as part of the Protomedicato, the royal licensing board examining surgeons for licenses, he found "many with good abilities, who in lacking books in their own language, were very far behind in what they could know."[2] The use and justification of the vernacular for a learned text were just two of the innovations Daza Chacón and other surgeons offered in their texts. It is notable, however, that those justifications were grounded in tradition—references to ancient and medieval authors. Indeed, the continuing influence of medieval authors is reflected in Daza Chacón's denigration of available translations of Guy de Chauliac and others, which he argues were not just difficult or rough in language, but dangerous in mistranslating the doctrines.[3] His unique combination of learning and skills enables him to not just translate what others have had to say, but to build on those medieval textual foundations while also offering innovation in format, content, language, and style.

Foundations

Sixteenth-century surgeons harked back to the medieval tradition not only by giving direct references to authors, including (most commonly) Guy de Chauliac (Guido), Bruno Longobucco (Bruno), Lanfranc of Milan (Lanfranco), William of

DOI: 10.4324/9781003291060-4

Saliceto (Guillermo de Saliceto), and Arnau of Villanova (Arnaldo) but also by writing texts that bore many parallels to those of their predecessors. Authors in both eras grounded their texts in references to ancient authorities while also incorporating new information. For medieval authors, the twelfth-century Renaissance brought new translations of surgical works by al-Rāzī (Rhazes), Ibn Sina (Avicenna), al-Zahrawi (Albucasis), and al-Majusi (Haly Abbas).[4] Similarly, fifteenth-century humanists sought out previously overlooked ancient texts while also offering new translations or editions of known texts. By the mid-sixteenth century, surgeons had access to not only a greater number of authors but also more translations (Latin, Greek, and vernacular) of texts. A key example is the Roman encyclopedist Celsus, whose medical text was discovered only in the 1420s and then became widespread with the first Latin printing in 1478. By the sixteenth century, Celsus, in various printed editions, had become a fundamental reference for all the authors considered here.[5]

Both medieval and Renaissance surgeons also actively sought to broaden the domain of surgery. Thirteenth-century surgeons incorporated discussions of conditions not addressed in ancient surgical texts, such as dropsy, cataracts, hernia, bladder stones, and scabies, much of which they based on information from Arabic texts combined with experience.[6] Renaissance surgeons likewise made a new effort to widen the scope of surgery, much of it based on personal experience. They incorporated urology, legal medicine, and plastic surgery, among other things. These new areas of expertise are discussed in more detail in Chapter 5.

While medieval medical texts were generally organized anatomically, from head to toe, surgical texts were more often structured around the type of ailments surgeons most often treated: wounds, tumors or swellings, fractures and dislocations.[7] Some authors included treatises on anatomy and medications as well. Medieval authors wrote for varying reasons—for students, to compile ancient authorities, to reconcile linguistic differences among those authorities, to show the learned nature of surgery.[8] Renaissance surgeons generally followed similar patterns, motivated to help students or other practitioners. As discussed in more detail in this chapter, they also had individual motivations and interests that shaped their approach to writing and what they included. Most commonly, Spanish surgeons organized their treatises by ailments, discussing tumors, wounds, and ulcers.

One Renaissance text, that of Bartolomé Hidalgo de Agüero, has a more direct resonance as a continuation of medieval texts. In his *Tesoro*, Hidalgo de Agüero advocated for a "new" method of healing, one with the least intervention in wounds possible. Hidalgo de Agüero traced these ideas back to Galen, who describes them being used by others though not by himself, and only for certain kinds of head wounds. Hidalgo de Agüero then acknowledges that he has built on the work of previous medieval surgeons, including Teodorico (d. 1296/8) and Nicolo Florentino (Niccolò Falcucci, d. 1412), who set forth similar principles of healing. Indeed, medieval historians have traced a similar line of thinking from the late thirteenth century through Henri de Mondeville in the fourteenth. Mondeville's text was left unfinished at his death, however, and this "dry" system of healing, which advocated against cautery of wounds or moist bandaging, was subsequently rejected by Guy de Chauliac whose 1363 *Chirurgia magna* reached greater heights of influence. Hidalgo de Agüero does not mention any of these French authorities, he simply argues that earlier writers provided only fragmented pieces, a sort of base to work from. In his account, only he has fully developed both the theory and practice, tested it over time, and given it a name, the *vía particular*.[9]

Finally, authors in both eras sought authority in language, though here we find a divergence. Medieval medical writers used Latin as the language of scholarship. It was the language of the ancient sources and remained the language of intellectual authority, whether theological or academic. The authors of twelfth-century surgical texts wrote not just to pass on information, but also to raise the intellectual status of surgery, applying theory and raising it on par with physic.[10] Whether written from within or outside of universities, medieval texts used writing, and in particular Latin writing, to signify learning beyond mere craft. The shift to vernacular languages in many disciplines from the fifteenth century on included medicine as well as science.[11] This linguistic shift happened slowly and certainly not without debate, but in the sixteenth century, it was increasingly common to find Latin texts translated into the vernacular, but also vernacular texts then translated into Latin, as was the case with Nicolas Monardes and Francisco Arceo.[12] Though some learned surgeons such as Giovanni da Vigo and Giovanni Andrea della Croce, published texts in both Latin and Italian, Spanish surgeons chose either Latin or Castilian.[13] An exception is Juan Fragoso, though he used Latin only for botanical treatises and Castilian for surgical ones.

Language and Authority

The growth of vernacular scientific and medical texts throughout Europe, whether original compositions or in translation from Latin or Greek, has received much attention.[14] The term vernacular medicine, however, has come to have multiple meanings. Recent studies have used vernacular to refer not just to the language used but also to genres of writing aimed at a general or non-professional audience. In this second use, vernacular stands in for popular, another term with variable and complex meanings.[15] Scholars examining vernacular or popular medical texts have recognized a different purpose, audience, and presentation from academic texts. These texts, including regimen books, recipe collections, books of secrets, and plague treatises had an audience that ranged from nobles to literate merchants and artisans, all seeking health advice.[16] Sandra Cavallo, in her study of medical advice books in Italy, explains vernacular as referring not only to language but also "to the accessible manner in which medical information was presented, both at textual level and in visual form."[17] She argues that many popular texts appealed to a nonacademic audience through the format of the text itself—line spacing, typography, page layout, and use of images. The visual accessibility of these texts matched the linguistic accessibility.

Although some surgical authors, such as the German Heironymus Brunschwig, wrote specifically for the "common man," the majority of vernacular surgical texts had a more limited audience.[18] In his comparison of late medieval vernacular translations of Teodorico's "Chirurgia" and Arnau de Vilanova's "Regimen Sanitatis," Cifuentes finds evidence of this divide: the audience for surgical texts was surgeons, while the audience for regimen texts was more general.[19] The same held true for Renaissance vernacular surgical texts. They were vernacular in language, not in content, and written for medical practitioners, not the "sickly reader" described by Solomon.[20] Instead of rhetoric meant to convince patients of efficacy or legitimacy, they offered rhetoric meant to convince practicing surgeons of the validity of the knowledge they offered, often a combination of ancient theory and modern empiricism.

Traditionally, the growing body of vernacular surgical texts in France, Germany, and Italy has been taken as emblematic of a new kind of surgeon: a highly skilled empirical practitioner who rose to prominence and was literate though not Latinate. Surgeons like Ambroise Paré and Thomas Vicary learned by doing and improved their skills by trial and error, gaining recognition and eventually positions at the French and English courts. While they had no choice but to write in the vernacular, their authority rested in the success they had achieved rather than in the language used. This overlooks the learned surgeons, for whom the vernacular was a deliberate choice, made to accommodate the limitations of the audience not the limitations of the author. Spanish surgeons who wrote in the vernacular often used the term *romance* in much the same way as vernacular—it referred to both the romance language of Castilian and when used as an adjective (*romancista*) implied someone non-Latinate and therefore less learned. Surgical texts *en romance*, however, were not aimed at a general audience. They retained the structure and presentation of academic works, not popular ones. They were replete with prefatory materials including approvals or endorsements of medical authorities, laudatory sonnets, and long dedicatory letters often filled with allusions to classical literature and Latin phrases. Most also then have prologues addressed to the reader which further signal their intended audience of medical students or practitioners. The texts themselves are written in dense prose, often printed in double columns with frequent marginal notes referring to other texts. Several of these texts are in two or more parts, each part consisting of four to six books and each book composed of anywhere from seven to fifty chapters. Unlike many other surgical texts (learned as well as popular) from other parts of Europe, there are no images in most of them, with the exception of a few drawings of instruments (see Figures 4.2 and 5.2).

Of the nine Spanish surgeons studied here, two insisted on writing in Latin in order to restrict their readership to educated elites. That Andrés Alcázar published in Latin is no surprise, as he was the only fully academic surgeon. As the inaugural professor of surgery at the University of Salamanca, he composed the *Chirurgiae libri sex* (1575) for his students and for posterity. Focused on training the new generation of university-educated surgeons, he had no interest in a broader audience of romance surgeons. His six books on surgery follow the medical head-to-toe format, though in this case, it is just head-to-lower abdomen. The first four books discuss injuries to the head, nerves, thorax, and lower abdomen, while the last two books examine morbo gálico and plague. Interestingly, Alcázar's is one of the few Spanish surgical texts to contain a few images, something more often associated with vernacular texts (in both senses of the word). In discussing head wounds, he includes several small illustrations, each showing a head in profile with bladed weapons causing wounds from different angles (see Figure 4.1).[21] He also includes some illustrations of instruments, particularly of trepans demonstrating improvements he made that made them easier to use and safer for the patient (see Figure 4.2).[22]

The other defender of Latin for surgical texts was Francisco Arceo. His 1574 text, *De recta curandorum vulnerum ratione*, begins with his reasoning against using the vernacular. This medical knowledge was powerful, but dangerous in uneducated hands. For Arceo, the ability to understand Latin was a measure of one's intellectual readiness to use this knowledge wisely. This argument is more intriguing as some scholars have questioned Arceo's own abilities in Latin, arguing that the linguistics of the text were heavily influenced by his friend and former student, Benito Arias Montano. Arias Montano had studied privately with Arceo during a time when he stayed with him. He presumably was among those who encouraged Arceo to write his text and wrote a preface for it, lauding Arceo's knowledge and skill. Benito Arias Montano was interested in many kinds of knowledge, but not in practicing medicine or surgery. He went on to gain international fame as a humanist, theologian, and natural philosopher.[23] By some historians' analysis, he likely also either wrote or at least edited the eloquent Latin in which the text is written.[24] It may be best, therefore, to treat this text as a joint effort of content from Arceo and style from Arias Montano. In addition, Arias Montano was instrumental in the publication work itself, bringing the work to the Plantin Press in Antwerp where he was connected both professionally and personally. Plantin's press was a hub of scientific printing in the sixteenth century, producing numerous works in various vernaculars as well as Latin. As a result, Arceo's text received international attention and was later translated into versions in English, Dutch, and German. Given the effort to which Arceo and Arias Montano went to polish and defend its Latin presentation, it seems all the more ironic that publication in Antwerp resulted in multiple vernacular renderings. Arceo's argument for Latin reflects the tensions that remained for learned authors, even as the vernacular became common for a variety of scientific and medical texts throughout Europe. In the Iberian Peninsula, however, the turn to the vernacular for many disciplines was not new.

The Iberian vernaculars of Castilian and Catalan gained impetus from the translation movement of the twelfth century. The perpetually contested political divisions of the Iberian Peninsula had created a medieval patchwork of populations who practiced various religions (Christian, Muslim, and Jewish) and who spoke or wrote multiple dialects including not only Latin, Castilian, Catalan, Portuguese, Hebrew, and Arabic but also linguistic hybrids such as Aljamiado (romance languages written in Arabic script), Ladino (Judeo-Spanish) and Mozarabic (Andalusi Romance). The early translation movement, which sought to render Arabic works into Latin, gained momentum and support in Toledo a half century after its conquest by the forces of Alfonso VI of Castile in 1085. The city had already been an important intellectual center, with some emphasis on scientific (particularly astronomical) knowledge while under the control of the Banū Dhul-Nun during the era of Taifa Kingdoms (1035–85).[25] The relatively nonviolent political change that brought Alfonso VI control over the city left intact a diverse general population of Muslims, Jews, and Christians, and particularly of Mozarabs or "Arabized" Christians fluent in Arabic as well as Castilian. It also left intact libraries and text collections. Thus, by the mid-twelfth century, both foreign and local scholars had begun to arrive in Toledo to access the knowledge available in Arabic texts. Most famous among those translators was Gerard of Cremona, drawn to Toledo in search of Ptolemy's *Almagest*, who then remained in the city translating a vast corpus of other works as well. Though Gerard's name is one that can be readily attached to numerous translations, it is clear that he worked with many others given the range and breadth of topics translated. Best known among the local Spaniards working alongside Gerard was Dominicus Gundissalinus, Archdeacon of Cuéllar but resident in Toledo.[26] Local Mozarabs were often key contributors, providing intermediary translations from Arabic to local dialects, which were then further refined into Latin.[27] The multinational nature of the translation movement has received the most attention from scholars, at the expense of recognizing Iberian contributions and dispersals.[28]

The most significant boost in the formalization of the Castilian language came in the next century, under the reign of Alfonso X (r. 1252–84), commonly known as *el Sabio* (the learned) for his patronage of scholarship on a wide range of topics. Alfonso is credited with fostering the earliest work on language formation in Castilian, sponsoring the production of the first vernacular law code, the *Siete Partidas*, and composing his own poetry and prose.[29] As Burns has aptly summed up, Alfonso's determination to promote Castilian over Latin prompted him to have a wide variety of texts, "scientific, literary, historical, juridical, and other works, both originals and translations, put into Castilian."[30] Castilian became the language of law and government as well as learning and culture in thirteenth-century Castile.

From the twelfth century on, then, literate medical practitioners in Iberia had access to vernacular manuscript translations of both ancient and Arabic medical texts. This vernacular tradition continued and expanded in the following centuries as scholars produced new vernacular translations of late medieval Latin authors including Lanfranc, Henri de Mondeville, Bernard of Gordon, and Guy de Chauliac.[31]

By the end of the fifteenth century, most of these texts were printed as well, at presses in Seville, Toledo, Salamanca, and Burgos. Recent work on the history of publishing in the sixteenth century has shown that in both Spain and Portugal, the vernacular continued to flourish in the printing presses, whose aggregate output in Latin over the course of the century remained just under 30%. This was not to say that the study and use of Latin were low, merely that Latin texts were predominantly imported rather than published in Iberia.[32] Thus, the flourishing of vernacular surgical texts in Spain was simply a continuation of a long tradition.

Still, the choice of language remained an issue to be addressed. Those who wrote in Castilian continued to explicitly justify its use in a learned text, while those who wrote in Latin argued it was preferable to keep such technical learning restricted to the truly learned. In defending the vernacular, authors insisted it was the knowledge that mattered rather than the form. Education and learning were reflected in concepts or ideas, not simply in the language one chose. Juan Calvo argues that he writes, "imitating the Ancients, most of whom wrote in their own languages."[33] Daza Chacón, in the prologue of one of his treatises, first quotes Hippocrates, arguing that "the patient looks for remedy, not language," and then follows this with his own statement that "what is needed is to understand the situation, know the ailment and quickly apply the remedy, and these one can do in whatever language they prefer." [34]

In addition, Spanish surgeons addressed the question of language and learning by reassuring their readers that writing in the vernacular was a conscious choice made by a learned practitioner. Juan Calvo states, "[T]he principal motivation for me to publish this has been the many requests made by surgeons, and because many of them do not read Latin, I have published this in the vernacular."[35] Juan Fragoso, most directly addresses the ongoing changes in surgical education, stating, "I published this work in Castilian because although the recent royal decree obliges surgeons to be Latinate and physicians, many are not."[36] Somewhat less directly, Hidalgo de Agüero provides a short glossary of terms at the beginning of his text, explaining that he found it necessary to use some terms from both Greek and Latin, explaining, "So that vernacular surgeons and others who are interested can easily enjoy this text it seemed to me important to help smooth the difficulties of some obscure terminology."[37]

The act of bridging Latin and vernacular medical cultures was not unique to surgeons, nor were the justifications they used for doing so.[38] Paula de Vos found a gradual decrease in Latin pharmacopoeias in the seventeenth century, replaced by Castilian. Authors address the same question of why they have written in the vernacular, using many of the same justifications of utility and practicality for those not trained in Latin. Whether these justifications for choosing the vernacular over Latin were defensive or had simply become an expected formality in print texts by the late sixteenth century is not clear, but they reflect the shifting intellectual context in which surgeons wrote and the continued connections of language and learning. The irony, of course, is that moving from Latin to vernacular made these texts accessible to a wider readership within Spain but less accessible to colleagues elsewhere. Several of these texts acquired a larger international audience only once they had been translated into Latin and disseminated either in that form or subsequently translated into other vernaculars. Regardless of the language chosen, however, all learned surgeons found their individual voices and shaped their texts in unique ways.

In their texts, Spanish surgeons most commonly address a standard set of bodily ailments: *apostemas* (tumors or swellings), *llagas* (fresh wounds, also known as *heridas nuevos*), and *úlceras* (old wounds or *llagas viejas*). Many, though not all, also include *fracturas* (fractures) and *dislocaciones* (dislocations). In some cases, such as in Dionisio Daza Chacón's *Practica y teorica* (1584), authors revert to the head-to-toe format within a category, discussing, for example, wounds to the head, neck, thorax, and so on down the body. Several include a treatise on anatomy (Fragoso, Calvo, Díaz), while others include an antidotary, or recipes for simple and compound remedies (Arceo, Fragoso, Hidalgo de Agüero). Beyond this, however, the texts all have unique aspects: Andrés de León's second book is a lengthy discussion of the soul; Francisco Arceo includes a chapter on cancer of the breast; Francisco Díaz's final book discusses four physical ailments surgeons should know how to cure: hemorrhoids, hernia, impetigo (as a general term for skin eruption), and *nimphea* (a protrusion of tissue from female genitalia).

Francisco Arceo's treatise includes a unique discussion of treating clubfoot in children.

> It sometimes happens that a child is born with one or both feet twisted, curved or flat, so that the child can hardly walk properly. So I want to describe a method that I have used to treat many very lame people, one of whom was a neighbor in Llerena who was difficult to treat, yet who finally regained his health by way of the method that I shall explain.[39]

Arceo's inclusion of this chapter is striking for several reasons. First, it was an unusual condition to be included in a surgical text, and this particular chapter sits a bit awkwardly in a text mostly focused on head wounds. This chapter, which includes detailed instructions on an orthopedic boot he developed, was added as an unnumbered chapter at the end of the second part.[40] In addition, the discussion of this condition stands out because it gives rise to the only illustration of the text, an outline drawing of the boot and frame Arceo developed to treat it. The image itself is not inserted into the text but comes at the end, which is a similarly awkward placement. While the earliest medical references to clubfoot seem to be from Hippocrates, it was not a condition addressed in later medical literature, and it seems to have become relegated to the work of bonesetters or other empirics, if it was treated at all. The third reason this discussion is interesting is because Arceo was not, in fact, alone in his discussion of clubfoot. Ambroise Paré also mentions it in his treatise, *Livre des monstres et Prodiges* (1573), but offers no treatment for it. Arceo medicalizes the condition, while Paré simply objectifies it, placing it among other malformations and "monstrosities." Paré does address treatment for clubfoot in later works, particularly in his collected works published in 1585. What inspired both men to turn their attention to this particular condition at roughly the same time is unclear, for neither mentions any reason for their discussion other than experience. Nonetheless, Arceo (followed by Paré) successfully moved treatment for clubfoot out of the realm of "unlearned" practitioners and added it to the list of those addressed by surgeons and for which their expertise was needed.

Print Culture

When Bartolomé Hidalgo de Agüero published his first work in 1584, it was not a weighty surgical manual composed of multiple books and chapters, but instead a simple broadsheet. He had been working at the Hospital del Cardinal in Seville for over two decades by that point and was renowned as both a healer and teacher. The broadsheet, titled "Avisos Particulares de Syrugia contra la Comun Opinion" (Propositions on Surgery Contrary to Current Views), listed forty-nine theses or propositions of surgical advice relating mostly to wound treatment (see Figure 3.1). The specific advice it contained (rejecting common approaches) and the accessibility of this short, printed sheet (written in the vernacular) prompted Dr. Estrada, a médico y cirujano visiting from Madrid, to make a formal protest to the city council. Estrada argued that much of Hidalgo de Agüero's advice was not simply contrary to common practice, but in fact dangerous to public welfare. He was also upset that Hidalgo de Agüero had written in the vernacular rather than Latin, which Estrada declared someone truly learned would not do.[41] Along with his letter of complaint, Estrada included his own explanatory refutation of several of the statements made by Hidalgo de Agüero, carefully explaining that he chose to also write in the vernacular only because that was the language originally used in the suspect treatise. Hidalgo de Agüero had the opportunity to respond to Estrada's challenge and defend his practices, both medical and linguistic. While there is no record of whether the two men ever conducted the experimental trials suggested by Estrada (in which each doctor would have one day to use his methods of healing on all patients who appeared for treatment at the hospital), Hidalgo de Agüero was clearly successful in defending his methods. He continued practicing and teaching at the Hospital del Cardenal and went on to write his more substantial text, which first reprinted the Avisos then went on to fully explain and defend them, complete with scholarly references.

This broadsheet was indeed an unusual publication for a learned surgeon. Similar ephemeral publications were extremely common for a wide range of purposes in sixteenth-century Europe, but not often preserved.[42] Like the vast majority (90%) of Spanish broadsheets surveyed by one study, only one known copy of this exists.[43] It is bound with Estrada's complaint and Hidalgo de Agüero's response in the volumes of city council records preserved in Seville's municipal archive. It is not clear why Hidalgo de Agüero had this sheet printed, nor how large the print run was. The format was also a common one for the sixteenth century, a series of theses with no further explanation. Similar printed broadsheets, known as *theses nudae* or bare theses, were used for medical students' university disputations in other parts of Europe in the sixteenth century. As Limbach's study of Basel has shown, however, such theses were generally circulated within the university system and were in Latin.[44] While there is no evidence for Hidalgo de Agüero holding a formal teaching position at the University of Seville, he did teach many students at the hospital, so it is possible this was meant to be used in a similar way to organize some sort of disputation with his students or among a broader medical community in Seville. He certainly succeeded in stirring up debate. Dr. Estrada responded almost immediately, but Juan Fragoso also saw this and published his own response and refutation to many of Hidalgo de Agüero's points, as discussed in the next chapter. In addition, the format of advertising a university disputation might help explain Dr. Estrada's

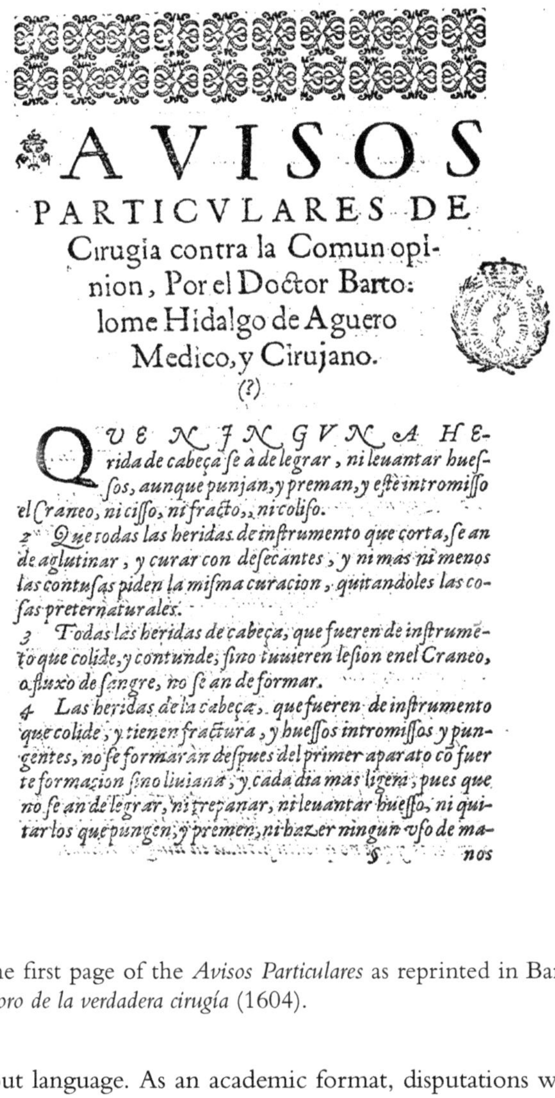

AVISOS
PARTICVLARES DE
Cirugia contra la Comun opi-
nion, Por el Doctor Barto:
lome Hidalgo de Aguero
Medico, y Cirujano.
(?)

QVE NINGVNA HE-
rida de cabeça se à de legrar, ni leuantar huessos, aunque punjan, y preman, y estè intromisso el Craneo, ni cisso, ni fracto, ni coliso.
2 Que todas las heridas de instrumento que corta, se an de aglutinar, y curar con desecantes, y ni mas ni menos las contusas piden la misma curacion, quitandoles las cosas preternaturales.
3 Todas las heridas de cabeça, que fueren de instrumẽto que colide, y contunde, sino tuuieren lesion enel Craneo, o fluxo de sangre, no se an de formar.
4 Las heridas de la cabeça, que fueren de instrumento que colide, y tienen fractura, y huessos intromissos y pungentes, no se formaràn despues del primer aparato cõ fuerte formacion sino liuiana, y cada dia mas ligera, pues que no se an de legrar, ni trepanar, ni leuantar huesso, ni quitarlos que pungen, y premen, ni hazer ningun vso de ma-
nos

FIGURE 3.1 The first page of the *Avisos Particulares* as reprinted in Bartolomé Hidalgo de Agüero, *Tesoro de la verdadera cirugía* (1604).

complaint about language. As an academic format, disputations were generally in Latin, and therefore, the published theses should also be written in Latin, not the vernacular. It is also possible, of course, that Hidalgo de Agüero had some other motivation for publishing. In any case, Hidalgo de Agüero's success in defending these ideas enabled him to write his much longer text, the *Tesoro de la verdadera cirugia*, which in the 1604 edition runs just over 290 folios. His text became just one of many, Latin and vernacular, that became available with each passing decade.

Renaissance surgeons were immersed in the world of print, which continued to expand over the course of the sixteenth century. The role of printing in disseminating knowledge to all levels of society, from the textbooks of university professors to the illustrated broadsides for the masses, has been well studied.[45] Printing of classical and medieval texts enabled medical students (and practitioners) to study a wide variety of authorities, while printed copies of the work of contemporaries enabled them to respond to new ideas as well, whether to embrace or reject them. Among the earliest ancient medical authors (who also addressed surgery) to be printed was Celsus, whose works in Latin appeared in 1478 and were frequently reprinted thereafter.[46] Certainly, Celsus was influential with all of the Spanish authors considered here, frequently cited throughout their texts.[47] Publication of additional ancient medical authors followed. In the first half of the sixteenth century, editions of the surgical works of Hippocrates (including, for example, an edition in Greek from the Aldine press in 1526 of *On Head Wounds*), Aëtius, and Oribasius were also published, making them better known and more widely available. Surgical works of Galen and Paul of Aegina also began to receive publication in the early sixteenth century, with rival Latin translations flourishing by mid-century.[48]

The types of medical works published in the sixteenth century expanded as well. Humanists began to read ancient texts more critically and to publish new forms of "error" literature, offering philological critiques of ancient works and their translations.[49] Other Latin texts focused on conflicting paradigms or controversial concepts from ancient authorities.[50] New genres of Latin medical writing included collections of medical letters, known as *epistolae medicae*, and collections of case studies, known as *observationes*.[51] As discussed earlier, vernacular medical texts also expanded in the fifteenth century, a trend that continued in the sixteenth. Along with the general works of regimen texts, recipe books, and disease treatises (plague and syphilis) aimed at the general literate public, came more focused texts on surgery, midwifery, and pharmacopoeia written for medical practitioners.[52]

While we have a good sense of the availability of printed texts, we have scant information on book ownership by Spanish learned surgeons. Dionisio Daza Chacón, whose father and uncle were both doctors, inherited books on medicine and surgery from his father, though the testament does not include an inventory, stating only that he should "take those that he wishes."[53] The only known personal library for a learned surgeon is that belonging to Francisco Díaz, who owned 146 medical books in Latin, Greek, and Castilian, as well as another fifty books on poetry, philosophy, and other topics.[54] Despite our lack of data on other learned surgeons, it is clear that they either owned or read enough to fill their own texts with references to specific passages from other works.

Printing enabled the wide circulation of these Spanish surgical texts, both within their lifetimes and in the century after. The text that eventually appeared throughout much of Europe was Arceo's *De recta curandorum vulnerum ratione*. The first Latin edition, published in Antwerp in 1574 and again in Amsterdam in 1658, was picked up by a wide range of scholars and eventually translated into multiple vernaculars with editions appearing in London (1588), Nuremberg (1600, 1674, 1717) Paris (1634), and Leeuwarden (1667). Within Spain, frequent reprintings, in multiple cities, of authors including Hidalgo de Agüero Calvo, Fragoso, Daza Chacón, and Pérez point to the widespread demand for these texts. These authors in particular were reprinted in cities in both Castile and Aragon: Calvo's *Primera y segunda parte de la cirugia universal y particular*, first printed in Seville (1580, 1598) was reprinted in Madrid (1626, 1657, 1674) and Valencia (1599, 1646, 1647, 1690, 1703); Fragoso's *Cirugía universal* had five printings in Madrid (1581, 1586, 1596, 1627, 1643, 1666), four in Alcalá (1592, 1601, 1607, 1621), and one in Zaragoza (1692); Daza Chacón's *Practica y teorica de cirugía en romance y latin* was printed four times in Valladolid (1585,1595, 1605, 1609) followed by three times in Madrid (1619, 1626, 1678) and twice in Valencia (1650, 1673); Pérez's *Suma y exámen de cirugía con breves esposiciones de algunas sentencias de Hipócrates y Galeno* underwent three editions in Madrid (1568, 1604, 1634), followed by Alcalá (1575), Zaragoza (1634), and Valencia (1634, 1649). Many of these works were also popular across the Atlantic in the colonies. The works of Calvo, Daza Chacón, Fragoso, Hidalgo de Agüero, Díaz, and de León have all been found among booksellers catalogues and in the inventories of libraries, both individual and institutional.[55] Printing enabled these learned surgeons to influence a wide range of practitioners across both time and space.

Bartolomé Hidalgo de Agüero's ability to overcome the concerns and complaints of Dr. Estrada demonstrates much of what made Renaissance learned surgeons stand out from their predecessors: new practices, challenges to traditional authorities, the use of print to disseminate ideas, and the extension of specialized knowledge to a broader vernacular audience. Learned surgeons claimed intellectual authority not only in their practices but also by composing texts that engaged with, embraced, revised, and at times outright rejected traditional theory and practices. More willing than their predecessors to rely on the authority of experience, they nonetheless carefully sought to use both ancient and medieval sources to bolster their new interpretations and practices. They took medieval texts as an authoritative template on which to build and then offered their own evidence of efficacy for what they changed. Taken as a whole, they changed a great deal. As the next chapters show, they refined the use of empiricism, the practices of wound treatment, and the use of (and tools for) trepanation. They expanded the surgeon's expertise to include urology, forensic medicine, and the treatment of diseases including plague, typhus, and morbo gálico. They incorporated and disseminated a wealth of other information on a number of other practices as well, from plastic surgery to treating aneurysms. Using the tripartite sources of ancient knowledge, medieval intellectual forms, and their own experiences, they sought to reshape this skilled and learned profession.

Notes

1 "Antes de que te de cuenta de mis trabajos y perigraciones (discreto Letor) te quiero dezir la occasion que me movió a escrivir en nuestra lengua Española, antes que en latina, que cierto a mi me fuera muy mas facil sin comparacion, y menos trabajo hazerlo en esta mas que en aquella: y la razon es evidentissima, porque si escriviera en latin no fuera necessario buscar la propria interpretacion del vocablo que usan los Cirujanos, ni traduzir los textos de los antiguos, y modernos, que me ha sido de grandissimo trabajo, sino pusieralos en el latin que ellos lo pusieron." Dionisio Daza Chacón, *Practica y teorica de cirugia en romance y en latin* (Valladolid: en casa de Ana Velez, 1609), Prologo al lector (n.p.).

2 "[V]i muchos que tenian muy buenas habilidades, que por falta de no tener libros en su lengua estavan muy atras de lo que pudieran saber" Daza Chacón, Prologo al lector (n.p.).

3 "Porque las traduciones de Guido y otros libros que se traen entre las manos, ha demas que la aspereca del lenguaje y poca fidelidad del interprete, hazen dubdosa y peligrosa la doctrina": Daza Chacón (1673), Epistola nuncupatoria al Lector (n.p).

4 Nancy G. Siraisi, "How to Write a Latin Book on Surgery: Organizing Principles and Authorial Devices in Guglielmo Da Saliceto and Dino Del Garbo," in *Practical Medicine from Salerno to the Black Death*, ed. Luis García Ballester et al. (New York: Cambridge University Press, 1994), 40.

5 Pedro Conde Parrado, "«Por el orden de Celso»: Aspectos de la influencia del De medicina en la cirugía europea del Renacimiento," *Dynamis: Acta Hispanica ad Medicinae Scientiarumque Historiam Illustrandam* 28 (2008): 217–42.

6 Michael R. McVaugh, *The Rational Surgery of the Middle Ages*, Micrologus' Library 15 (Firenze: SISMEL-Edizione del Galluzzo, 2006), Chapter 4.

7 Luke E. Demaitre, *Medieval Medicine: The Art of Healing, from Head to Toe* (Santa Barbara, CA: Praeger, 2013).

8 McVaugh, *The Rational Surgery of the Middle Ages*, 9–11; Siraisi, "How to Write a Latin Book on Surgery," 42–7.

9 Bartolomé Hidalgo de Agüero, *Thesoro de la verdadera cirugía y vía particular contra la común* (Sevilla: Francisco Pérez, 1604), fol. 81v. See also the fuller discussion of this in Chapter 4.

10 McVaugh, *The Rational Surgery of the Middle Ages*, 13–16.

11 William Crossgrove, "The Vernacularization of Science, Medicine, and Technology in Late Medieval Europe: Broadening Our Perspectives," *Early Science and Medicine* 5, no. 1 (2000): 47–63 provides a summary conclusion to the series of articles in *Early Science and Medicine* III (1998) and IV (1999).

12 Peter Burke, "Translations into Latin in Early Modern Europe," in *Cultural Translation in Early Modern Europe*, ed. Peter Burke and R. Po-chia Hsia (Cambridge: Cambridge University Press, 2007), 65–80, https://doi.org/10.1017/CBO9780511497193.005; Valerie Worth-Stylianou, "Concurrent Publication of Medical Works in Neo-Latin and French in Early Modern France," *Canadian Review of Comparative Literature/Revue Canadienne de Littérature Comparée* 41, no. 4 (2014): 456–76, https://doi.org/10.1353/crc.2014.0040; Ted Brown, "Word Wars: The Debate over the Use of the Vernacular in Medical Writings of the English Renaissance," *Texas Studies in Literature and Language* 37, no. 1 (1995): 98; Lluis Cifuentes, "Vernacularization as an Intellectual and Social Bridge. the Catalan Translations of Teodorico's Chirurgia and of Arnau De Vilanova's Regimen Sanitatis," *Early Science & Medicine* 4, no. 2 (May 1999): 127; Erwin Huizenga, "Unintended Signatures: Middle Dutch Translations of Surgical Works," in *Science Translated: Latin and Vernacular Translations of Scientific Treatises in Medieval Europe*, ed. Michèle Goyens, Pieter de Leemans, and An Smets, Mediaevalia Lovaniensia, ser. 1, studia 40 (Leuven: Leuven University Press, 2008).

13 See the excellent study of della Croce's use of both languages by Cynthia Klestinec, "Translating Learned Surgery," *Journal of the History of Medicine and Allied Sciences* 72, no. 1 (2017): 34–50.

14 There is a vast bibliography on this topic. Recent studies are found in a special issue of *Nuncius* 36, no. 2 (2021). A sampling of scholarship for different languages would include Brown, "Word Wars"; Howard Stone, "The French Language in Renaissance Medicine," *Bibliothèque d'Humanisme et Renaissance* 15, no. 3 (1953): 315–46; Irma Taavitsainen and Päivi Pahta, "Vernacularisation of Scientific and Medical Writing in Its Sociohistorical Context," in *Medical and Scientific Writing in Late Medieval English*, ed. Irma Taavitsainen and Päivi Pahta, Studies in English Language (New York: Cambridge University Press, 2004), 1–19; Caroline Boucher and Geneviève Dumas, "Traductions et Compilations Médicales: Une Coïncidence Obligée?," *Early Science and Medicine* 17, no. 3 (2012): 273–308, https://doi.org/10.1163/157338212X645094; Karine van't Land, "'Because My Son Does Not Read Latin' Rhetoric, Competition and Education in Middle Dutch Surgical Handbooks,'" *Studies in Ancient Medicine* 35 (2010): 443–59.

15 Bob Scribner, "Is a History of Popular Culture Possible?," *History of European Ideas* 10, no. 2 (January 1, 1989): 175–91, https://doi.org/10.1016/0191-6599(89)90067-3; Sabrina Minuzzi, "Printing Medical Knowledge: Vernacular Genres, Reception and Dissemination," *Nuncius* 36, no. 2 (June 23, 2021): 193–97, https://doi.org/10.1163/18253911-03602015.
16 Paul Slack, "Mirrors of Health and Treasures of Poor Men: The Uses of Vernacular Medical Literature of Tudor England," in *Health, Medicine and Mortality in the Sixteenth Century*, ed. Charles Webster (New York: Cambridge University Press, 1979), 237–73; William Eamon, *Science and the Secrets of Nature: Books of Secrets in Medieval and Early Modern Culture* (Princeton, NJ: Princeton University Press, 1994); Tillmann Taape, "Common Medicine for the Common Man: Picturing the 'Striped Layman' in Early Vernacular Print," *Renaissance Quarterly* 74, no. 1 (2021): 1–58, https://doi.org/10.1017/rqx.2020.315; Sandra Cavallo, "Early Vernacular Medical Advice Books and Their Popular Appeal in Early Modern Italy," *Nuncius* 36, no. 2 (2021): 264–303, https://doi.org/10.1163/18253911-03602003; Elaine Leong, "Learning Medicine by the Book: Reading and Writing Surgical Manuals in Early Modern London," *BJHS Themes* 5 (2020): 93–110, https://doi.org/10.1017/bjt.2020.7.
17 Cavallo, "Early Vernacular Medical Advice Books and Their Popular Appeal in Early Modern Italy," 265.
18 Taape, "Common Medicine for the Common Man."
19 Cifuentes, "Vernacularization as an Intellectual and Social Bridge. the Catalan Translations of Teodorico's "Chirurgia" and of Arnau De Vilanova's "Regimen Santitatis.""
20 Michael Solomon, *Fictions of Well-Being: Sickly Readers and Vernacular Medical Writing in Late Medieval and Early Modern Spain* (Philadelphia: University of Pennsylvania Press, 2010).
21 Andrés Alcázar, *Andreae Alcazaris Medici, ac Chirurgi Guadalaxarensis in amplissima Salmanticensi Academia Chirurgae facultatis primi Professoris Chirurgiae libri sex: in quibus multa antiquorum, et recentiorum sub obscura loca hactemus non declarata interpretantur* (Salamanca, 1575), 21–2.
22 Alcázar, *Chirurgiae libri sex* trepans are shown pp. 62–4; other instruments are illustrated on 150, 151,153, 161.
23 María M. Portuondo, *The Spanish Disquiet: The Biblical Natural Philosophy of Benito Arias Montano* (Chicago: The University of Chicago Press, 2019).
24 Enrique Montero Cartelle, "Benito Arias Montano y Francisco Arceo: la Redacción del *De recta curandorum vulnerum ratione*," *Asclepio* 64, no. 2 (2012): 417–34, https://doi.org/10.3989/asclepio.2012.v64.i2.527.
25 Charles Burnett, "The Coherence of the Arabic-Latin Translation Program in Toledo in the Twelfth Century," *Science in Context* 14, no. 1–2 (2001): 249–50.
26 Burnett, "The Coherence of the Arabic-Latin Translation Program in Toledo in the Twelfth Century"; Marie-Therese d'Alverny, "Translations and Translators," in *Renaissance and Renewal in the Twelfth Century*, ed. Robert Louis Benson et al. (Cambridge, MA: Harvard University Press, 1982), 452–4.
27 Burnett, "The Coherence of the Arabic-Latin Translation Program in Toledo in the Twelfth Century," 252.
28 d'Alverny, "Translations and Translators."
29 Herbert Allen Van Scoy and Ivy A. Corfis, *A Dictionary of Old Spanish Terms Defined in the Works of Alfonso X* (Madison: Hispanic Seminary of Medieval Studies, 1986); Lloyd Kasten, "Alfonso El Sabio and the Thirteenth-Century Spanish Language," in *Emperor of Culture: Alfonso X the Learned of Castile and His Thirteenth-Century Renaissance*, ed. Robert Ignatius Burns (Philadelphia: University of Pennsylvania Press, 1990), 33–45.
30 Robert I. Burns, S.J., ed., "Stupor Mundi: Alfonso X of Castile, the Learned," in *Emperor of Culture: Alfonso X the Learned of Castile and His Thirteenth-Century Renaissance* (Philadelphia: University of Pennsylvania Press, 1990), 9.
31 Luis S. Granjel, *Cirugía Española Del Renacimiento* (Salamanca: Universidad de Salamanca, 1968), 21–4.

32 Alexander S. Wilkinson, ed., *Iberian Books/Libros ibéricos (IB): Books Published in Spanish or Portuguese or on the Iberian Peninsula before 1601/Libros publicados en español o portugués o en la Península Ibérica antes de 1601* (Boston: Brill, 2010), xviii–xix.

33 "[I]mitando a los Antiguos, que los mas escrivian sus obras en sus proprias lenguas" Juan Calvo, *Primera y segunda parte de la cirugia uniuersal y particular del cuerpo humano* (Madrid: Diego Flamenco, 1626), Prologo.

34 "[E]l enfermo no busca lenguas, sino remedio"; "lo que hace al caso es entender el negocio, y conocer la enfermedad, y aplicarle a tiempo el conveniente remedio, y esto sea en la lengua que quisiere." Dionisio Daza Chacón, *Pratica y teorica de cirugia en romance y en latin* (por Francisco Cipres, 1673), 175.

35 "[E]l principal intento que me a movido a imprimirlo, ha sido, porque muchas vezes me lo han rogado los Cirujanos: y como estos por la mayor parte son Romancistas, por esso se ha impresso en romance" Juan Calvo, *Primera y segunda parte de la cirugia uniuersal y particular del cuerpo humano* (Madrid, 1674), Prologo.

36 "saque a luz este libro en el vulgar Castellano: porque aunque es verdad que la nueva prematica oblige a los Cirujanos a ser Latinos y Medicos ay muchos Romancistas." Juan Fragoso and Francisco Díaz, *Cirugia vniuersal, aora nueuamenta añadida…: Iten otros quatro tratados, el primero es vna suma de proposiciones contra auisos de cirugia, el segundo de las declaraciones acerca de diuersas heridas y muertes, el tercero, de los Aphorismos de Hipocrates tocantes a cirugia, el cuarto, de la naturaleza y calidades de los medicamentos simples; Iten vn tratado de todas las enfermedades de los riñones, vexiga y carnosidades de la verga y orina y de su cura…; por Francisco Diaz…* (por la viuda de Alonso Martin, 1627), Al Lector (n.p.).

37 Hidalgo de Agüero, *Tesoro*. This alphabetical listing of terms, two-pages long, follows an eight-page listing of the table of contents.

38 Michela Pereira, "Alchemy and the Use of Vernacular Languages in the Late Middle Ages," *Speculum* 74, no. 2 (April 1999): 336–56, https://doi.org/10.2307/2887050; Paula De Vos, "Pharmacopoeias and the Textual Tradition in Galenic Pharmacy," in *Drugs on the Page: Pharmacopoeias and Healing Knowledge in the Early Modern Atlantic World*, ed. Matthew James Crawford and Joseph M. Gabriel (Pittsburgh, PA: University of Pittsburgh Press, 2019), 19–44.

39 José Ramón Vallejo, Marina Mesa, and José M Cobos-Bueno, "Francisco Arceo de Fregenal and the Treatment of Clubfoot up to the Sixteenth Century," *Acta Medico-Historica Adriatica* 16, no. 1 (2018): 33, https://doi.org/10.31952/amha.16.1.1.

40 Francisco Arceo, *De recta curandorum vulnerum ratione et aliis eius artis praeceptis libri II: eiusdem De febrium curandarum ratione* (ex officina Christophori Plantini, 1574), 167–72.

41 Archivo Municipal de Sevilla, Sección 3, Tomo 11, n. 75. "cosa no acostumbrado entre letrados."

42 Andrew Pettegree, ed., *Broadsheets: Single-Sheet Publishing in the First Age of Print* (Boston: Brill, 2017), http://brill.com/view/title/34448.

43 Alexander S. Wilkinson, Alejandra Ulla Lorenzo, and Alba de la Cruz, "A Survey of Printed Spanish Broadsheets, 1472–1700," in *Broadsheets: Single-Sheet Publishing in the First Age of Print*, vol. 60, Library of the Written Word (Brill, 2017), 55–75.

44 Saskia Limbach, "Advertising Medical Studies in Sixteenth-Century Basel: Function and Use of Academic Disputations," in *Broadsheets: Single-Sheet Publishing in the First Age of Print*, ed. Andrew Pettegree, vol. 60, Library of the Written Word (Leiden: Brill, 2017), 376–98.

45 The literature on printing is too vast to recount here. Eisenstein remains foundational, but her work has been challenged, refined, and expanded by Grafton, Maclean, Jones, Pettegree, and many others. For medical printing in particular see, among others, Stone, "The French Language in Renaissance Medicine"; Ian Maclean, *Logic, Signs and Nature in the Renaissance: The Case of Learned Medicine* (New York: Cambridge University Press, 2007); Ian Maclean, "The Diffusion of Learned Medicine in the Sixteenth Century through the Printed Book," in *Learning and the Market Place: Essays in the History of the Early Modern Book* (Boston: Brill, 2009); Laurence Brockliss and Colin Jones, *The Medical World of Early Modern France* (New York: Oxford University Press, 1997).

46 Vivian Nutton, "Humanist Surgery," in *The Medical Renaissance of the Sixteenth Century*, ed. A. Wear, R. K. French, and Iain M. Lonie (New York: Cambridge University Press, 2009), 77–8.
47 See also Ana I. Martín Ferreira, "El ideal de Celso en la cirugía española del s. XVI," *Medizinhistorisches Journal* 30, no. 2 (1995): 145–65; Conde Parrado, "«Por el orden de Celso»."
48 Vivian Nutton, "Humanist Surgery," in *The Medical Renaissance of the Sixteenth Century*, ed. A. Wear, R. K. French, and Iain M. Lonie (New York: Cambridge University Press, 2009), 77–9.
49 Maclean, *Logic, Signs and Nature in the Renaissance*, 18–22.
50 José María López Piñero and Francisco Calero, *Los temas polémicos de la medicina renacentista: Las "Controversias" (1556) de Francisco Valles* (Madrid: Consejo superior de investigaciones científicas, 1988); Gianna Pomata, "Sharing Cases: The *Observationes* in Early Modern Medicine," *Early Science and Medicine* 15, no. 3 (2010): 193–236, https://doi.org/10.1163/157338210X493932.
51 Nancy G. Siraisi, *Communities of Learned Experience: Epistolary Medicine in the Renaissance*, Singleton Center Books in Premodern Europe (Baltimore, MD: Johns Hopkins University Press, 2013); Gianna Pomata, "Observation Rising: Birth of an Epistemic Genre, 1500–1650," in *Histories of Scientific Observation*, ed. Lorraine Daston and Elizabeth Lunbeck (Chicago, IL: University of Chicago Press, 2011), 45–80; Pomata, "Sharing Cases."
52 Maclean, *Logic, Signs and Nature in the Renaissance*, 40–1; De Vos, "Pharmacopoeias and the Textual Tradition in Galenic Pharmacy," 39–40; Brockliss and Jones, *The Medical World of Early Modern France*, 98–9.
53 "[D]e los libros quel tiene de medizina y zurujia tome todos los quel quisiere" Anastasio Rojo Vega, "1575 Codicilo Del Doctor Bernardino Daza Chacón, Médico y Padre Del Licenciado Dionisio Daza | Real Biblioteca | Investigadores," Real Biblioteca Investigadores, accessed March 8, 2022, https://investigadoresrb.patrimonionacional.es/node/5714.
54 Emilio Maganto Pavón, "Francisco Díaz," Historia de la Urología Española, n.d., http://historia.aeu.es/FranciscoDiaz.htm; José Antonio Perálvarez, "Francisco Díaz, Padre de La Urología," *Historias de Alcalá* (blog), Publicado el agosto 2015, https://historiasdealcala.wordpress.com/2015/08/03/francisco-diaz-padre-de-la-urologia/.
55 Linda A. Newson and Susie Minchin, *From Capture to Sale: The Portuguese Slave Trade to Spanish South America in the Early Seventeenth Century*, The Atlantic World, v. 12 (Leiden; Boston: Brill, 2007), 267–9; Linda A. Newson, *Making Medicines in Early Colonial Lima, Peru: Apothecaries, Science and Society* (Boston: Brill, 2017), 131–7; Jose Torre Revello, *El libro, la imprenta y el periodismo en América durante la dominación española*, no. 74 (Buenos Aires: Publicaciones del Instituto de Investigaciones Historicas, 1940), 242; Carlos Alberto González Sánchez, Tristán Platt, and Bethany Aram, *New World Literacy: Writing and Culture across the Atlantic, 1500–1700*, The Bucknell Studies in Latin American Literature and Theory (Lewisburg: Lewisburg Bucknell University Press, 2011), 85, 177.

4

REFINING KNOWLEDGE AND PRACTICE

Empiricism, Tradition, and Innovation

Francisco Díaz begins the prologue to his *Compendio de chirurgia* (1575) as many did in this era, with an address to the reader and an explanation of his text: "You will find, inquisitive reader, in this treatise a compendium of surgery, divided in four books." After briefly listing the contents of the four books (anatomy, apostemas, fresh wounds, old wounds), as well as an additional short treatise on four "rare and dangerous conditions/ailments," he goes on to state his motivations for publishing it.

> Having seen the lack of books for surgeons without Latin…I have published this treatise with information from illustrious authors both Greek and Arabic…as also with the wide experience of many years of my own work in notable places of Spain, principally in the city of Burgos, where I had great success.[1]

Drawing upon his own experiences alongside the wisdom of Greek and Arabic authorities gave Díaz purpose for writing.

Renaissance surgeons, whether employing their skills on battlefields or in communities, participated in new forms of knowledge construction, based on both authority and experience. The humanism that brought forth new Greek and Latin editions of ancient authors, reestablishing the importance of these authorities and texts, also encouraged new interpretations of them (linguistic as well as practical) leading to new genres of critique and the disputation of errors.[2] The sixteenth century was a time of intellectual argument, debate, and upheaval. As the authority of ancients came into question, experience and observation gained greater respect.[3] In this way, learned surgeons embodied the Renaissance dichotomy of returning to ancient writings only to wrestle with which parts to embrace and which to challenge or reinterpret. Bartolomé Hidalgo de Agüero provides a good example of this process of fusing forms of knowledge. Writing in the 1580s, he advocated an alternate method of wound treatment, an approach he named the vía particular

DOI: 10.4324/9781003291060-5

in contrast to the traditional approach, which he named the vía comun. To support his argument for this new approach, he draws first from personal experience as a surgeon and then turns to ancient authority as a means of both showing his own erudition and bolstering the argument for his practices.

Hidalgo de Agüero first offers the authority of experience to establish his expertise:

> I can affirm as an eyewitness who has been healing for more than twenty years and held public positions at the Hospital del Cardenal in Seville and others… and having practiced the particular as well as the comun and having found such great benefit [from the former] that I have become obliged not only to practice it but also to share it.[4]

He then quantifies his success, attesting that in 1583, he had treated 456 wounded patients at the hospital, of whom only twenty had died. Narrowing his scope to focus only on head wounds and only in the previous two and a half months, he states fifty out of fifty-seven had been healed, with only seven dying. Finally, he provides a comparison (albeit much less numerically concrete) to the success of the standard method, asserting that "in the years in which my predecessors worked, and in which I also used the traditional method, more patients died than survived."[5]

After personal experience, Hidalgo de Agüero's second justification for his innovative treatment was to turn to Galen. This both established his own erudition and provided him a means of suggesting that this method was, in fact, *not* an innovation but based on ancient practice and had been described by Galen in positive terms. He gives reference to Book VI of Galen's *Method of Medicine* in a marginal note, though he does not quote the text directly. Examining the final passage of this text, we find Galen discussing the proper medicines and care after trepanation in head wounds:

> It just remains for me still to consider what the best form of medication is and the whole care after the trepanning. This is, whether it is the most mild and paregoric, as now used by the majority, or the complete opposite of this, by means of those medications that are very strongly drying—medications of the sort Meges the Sidonian also praises. And a fellow citizen of mine always used [drying medicines].… I have not seen anyone else use this, nor have I myself been brave enough to use it. This much only am I able to testify regarding Eudemus, for this was what the old man was called: that more of those people treated by him were saved than those who were treated with paregorics."[6]

Reading this passage, it becomes clear that Hidalgo de Agüero framed his own text much as Galen had: the use of the firsthand storytelling, the setting of a comparison between approaches to healing (paregoric vs. drying) in which the mild paregoric one is most commonly used and the drying is uncommon but clearly to be preferred, and the idea of quantifying (of a sort) the success rate of each as evidence in favor of the less used or less well-known approach. One might argue that Hidalgo de Agüero was simply being a true Renaissance scholar, returning to ancient sources and reviving a method Galen had already pointed to. But Galen also points out in this passage his own reluctance to ever try it himself, thus placing Hidalgo de Agüero in a position of contravening Galen's actual practices.

Hidalgo de Agüero's expertise in this matter rests on the dual platforms of book knowledge and personal experience, as well as his ability to explain how both kinds of knowledge bolster innovation. Despite these strategies of legitimizing new practices, many such innovations were challenged. Indeed, Hidalgo de Agüero quickly faced such challenges, in person from Dr. Estrada and in print from Juan Fragoso. Those disputes or challenges and responses to them were themselves important for further expanding and defining expertise and offer us a window into this process of amalgamating tradition, innovation, and experience.

Renaissance surgeons who developed new techniques and advocated for new practices did not propose any radically new overall theories about the body. The intellectual revolution they advocated was still based on the theory established and refined by ancient and medieval authors. They advocated for the importance of understanding humoral theory for treating the body, bolstering the surgeon's knowledge beyond what worked to *why* it worked. At the same time, learned surgeons offered practical innovations in instruments, methods or approaches, and therapeutic compounds. In the sixteenth century, the body and its structures were increasingly better understood thanks to the expansion of anatomical studies in the first half of the century, and beliefs about the humoral body and its balanced health were challenged by some but remained largely unchanged.

One exception was Paracelsus (1493–1541), the controversial advocate of an entirely new understanding of man and the natural world. Philippus Aureolus Theophrastus Bombastus von Hohenheim, better known by his adopted alias, Paracelsus, was a unique figure who rejected both ancient humoral theory and texts themselves as sources of knowledge. His promotion of chemical medicine certainly set him apart from most in his era, as did his reputation as a temperamental and often condescending practitioner and teacher.[7] But in advocating for empiricism and education based on the experience of the natural world and his rejection of the separation of physic and surgery, he was entirely in step with many other thinkers and writers of the time.[8] Many of Paracelsus's ideas and practices were controversial, but his work on surgery, *Dei grosse Wundarznei* (*Great Wound Surgery*, 1536) was translated into Latin and widely read.

The reception and influence of Paracelsus's writings (as well as those of his later followers) in Spain is a complicated one.[9] Paracelsus's works eventually appeared on the Spanish Index of Prohibited Books in 1583, when the Latin translation of his *Dei grosse Wundarznei*, known as *Chirurgia magna* (1573) was prohibited, while the *Chirurgia minor* (1570) required only some expurgation.[10] That Spaniards had access to these works both before and after expurgation is clear, as Francisco Díaz, Juan Fragoso, and Dionisio Daza Chacón all refer to him in their texts. However, no clear "Paracelsian" movement developed in Spain. In one of the later editions of his text, Juan Fragoso refers to the *Chirurgia magna* and quotes from Paracelsus's early critic Conrad Gesner, and he is quick to point out that he is working from an expurgated copy.[11] Paracelsus represents an extreme form of expertise based on experience or empiricism, which outright rejected prior knowledge. This certainly was not embraced by all, but Paracelsus's work is a useful reminder of how complicated the Renaissance embrace of empiricism was. Most sixteenth-century practitioners favored some combination of tradition and innovation, the latter driven by a new form of empiricism, but they continued to regard knowledge gained solely from "experience" with a measure of caution, if not disdain.

The challenge of balancing tradition and innovation was one of distinguishing valuable innovation from the dangerous dismissal of established practices. This was an era filled with debates over new ideas—Catholic and Protestant theologians debated new translations and interpretations of scripture, astronomers debated the reality versus practicality of Copernican heliocentrism, and medical men debated the new Vesalian anatomy. For surgeons, such debates were not just about doctrine, however. On a practical level, they held substantial, indeed mortal, consequences. Surgeons were in a unique position of straddling the theoretical and the practical, engaging in a range of disputes over theory and practice, based on both their book learning and their observations of cases. Sprinkled throughout these texts are references to their experiences with individual cases, evidence for expertise based on direct experience.

Medicine and Empiricism

To better understand the role of empiricism in Renaissance surgery, and particularly in the construction of knowledge and practices, it is helpful to examine the term and its applications over time. Medicine is an inherently empirical practice, for one needs to observe symptoms in order to diagnose and recommend treatment. While medieval and early modern physicians did not always observe patients firsthand—for example, they were at times brought urine from a patient by a third party for examination and diagnosis—they still relied upon their sensory observations of color, texture, and sedimentation of the urine to determine a diagnosis. The discussion of empiricism in medicine is further complicated by the term itself, which has held different meanings in different eras. While today it holds a positive connotation of association with modern science, in which experiment and observation hold a place of prominence, in the premodern era, it was defined more narrowly and at times viewed more skeptically or negatively.

The ancient Greek school of empiricism, one of many medical philosophies of that era, held an ideology of close observation of patients' symptoms while rejecting the utility of searching for (often hidden and therefore difficult to discern) causes. Instead, empirics advocated response to symptoms, which relied simply upon observation and the experience of what worked in the past without recourse to broader theories of health and remedies. Along with personal experience, then, came the recording of case histories to share successful cures. This created a movement of healers who, while eschewing analysis and theory, were nonetheless educated and text-based in their own way.[12] Galen himself trained with Empiricists, among others, and discusses the persuasiveness of many of their arguments.[13] Ultimately, for the ancient world, empiricism describes a way of thinking, an approach to knowledge that was based on the practical—what worked but not why it worked.[14] Opponents to this approach, such as Dogmatics, held theory as immensely superior to observation or experience and provide some of the earliest denigrations of "empirics."[15]

By the Renaissance, Empiricists had disappeared, but the term "empiric" was applied more loosely to a variety of healers, generally those with a narrow expertise gained by practice and little formal education in theory.[16] Considered part of the medical marketplace in medieval and early modern Europe, empirics encompassed a wide range of practitioners from the self-taught charlatan hawking fake remedies to apprentice-trained specialists whose experience enabled them to successfully treat particular conditions such as hernia, bladder stones, cataracts, or broken bones. Many were itinerant and unlicensed specialists, though others held surgical licenses and the line between "barber-surgeon" and empiric could be blurred to the point of invisibility.[17] In Spain, Philip II employed a number of empirics at his court, including Francisco and Diego de Somovilla (perhaps father and son), who were given specific charge for curing "stones, dislocations, and hernias."[18] Similarly, Diego Díaz specialized in urinary problems, while Alonso de Arce was employed specifically to set fractured or broken bones (*algebrista*).[19] Other early modern empirics offered "secret" remedies, proprietary compounds, and distillations, which they claimed would cure a variety of ailments. Arguably the most famous Spanish empiric of the sixteenth century was Aparicio de Zubia, whose famous healing oil brought him royal support from both Charles V and Philip II, as well as international recognition.[20] The growing recognition of empirics within the medical marketplace in the sixteenth century reflects the overall shift to a new appreciation of the value of experience. While modern definitions of empiricism link it to the use of experiment and the rise of modern science in the seventeenth century, scholars of Renaissance science have long recognized the roots of experimental science in the sixteenth century. The term "empiricism" retained a taint of illiteracy and ignorance in the sixteenth century, but the practices of experiment and observation, of trusting one's sensory perception, grew and flourished.

This new acknowledgment of experience underpinned the work of learned surgeons. As Andrés de León states outright, "[E]xperience is the mother of all things, and more essential than theory."[21] Yet learned surgeons were careful to frame their knowledge from experience with theory. Distancing themselves from both ancient Empiricists and modern empirics, these learned surgeons, including Dionisio Daza Chacón, Juan Fragoso, and Juan Calvo, began their texts with an overview of the ancient sects. Bartolomé Hidalgo de Agüero includes a lengthy (15 folios) treatise devoted to distinguishing seven different sects, ancient and modern, and how their methods would be applied in specific cases of wounds. In addition to discussing ancient sects, surgical authors cite a wide range of ancient authors, most often Hippocrates, Galen, Pliny, and Celsus. In so doing, these authors showed their knowledge of ancient theory, situating themselves as learned heirs of this past. Their texts offer a new practice of empiricism that melds the learned past with the experiential present.[22]

This new empiricism flourished not only in surgery but also in a variety of other related fields, including alchemy, botany, and anatomy. Like medicine, the roots of alchemical theories and practices can be traced to ancient times, waxing and waning in popularity over the centuries.[23] In the sixteenth century, alchemy flourished in a variety of forms at the courts of Europe, as well as across many cities.[24] Alchemists, concerned with a range of health topics, created medicinal distillations and infusions, oils, salves, and compounds. Books of secrets—compilations of both traditional and new remedies, recipes, and practical alchemy—flourished as well.[25] Sixteenth-century alchemical medicine has long been overshadowed by the larger-than-life figure of Paracelsus, but if we look beyond him, we find a range of alchemical practices, some linked to medicine and some not, flourishing throughout Europe.[26] Linking all forms of alchemy, as well as pharmacy and surgery, were notions of change and experiment. Experiment was key to finding the best way to elicit wanted changes, from the alchemical change of substance, to the cosmetic change of appearance, to the medical change of healing. In Spain, Philip II also provided extensive patronage to alchemists, who worked on a variety of projects, from the practical distillation of medicinal compounds to the ephemeral transmutation of metals to gold and the creation of potent elixirs.[27]

The new botanical empiricism arose from Europeans venturing to new lands both east and west, who brought or sent back new plants for food, spices, and medicine, all of which were tried, tasted, tested, and fit into existing botanical knowledge.[28] Across Europe, physicians with an interest in botany described and experimented with both domestic and foreign plants, from tomatoes (Pietro Andrea Mattioli) to tulips (Carolus Clusius) to tobacco (Nicolas Monardes), while others planted botanic gardens and experimented with the cultivation of exotic species. Successfully transplanting exotic seeds or shoots was difficult, as noted by Simón de Tovar, a physician and botanist in Seville, who recounted that

> with regard to the trees and shrubs from the Indies, they produce very few fruits in our soil. Those which do produce rarely bring their fruit to fruition, for they produce it so late and out of season that they lose their fruit before it is ripe under the first autumnal colds.[29]

Still, many persevered with varying success, and Seville became a center for experimental botany. Well-known botanic gardens were cultivated by Nicolas Monardes, Simón de Tovar, Hernando Colon, and Juan de Castañeda among others.[30]

European botanists, many trained in medicine, also began studying their local flora, expanding upon the ancient work of Dioscorides in efforts to name and describe not just medicinal plants but all other plants and their uses.[31] Recognizing the ancient texts as an important base of knowledge, the Italian physician and botanist Antonio Musa Brassavola pointed out the importance of current work for adding to that base, stating in his 1536 work, "Not a hundredth part of the herbs existing in the whole world was described by Dioscorides, not a hundredth part by Theophrastus or by Pliny, but we add more every day and the art of medicine advances."[32] Illustrated herbals provided new visual as well as textual descriptions. Several well-known botanists of the sixteenth century studied medicine and botany at mid-century at the University of Montpellier under Guillaume Rondelet, including Charles L'Ecluse (Clusius), Matthias de l'Obel (Lobelius), and Jacques Daleschamps, but botanists studied and published new texts in all areas of Europe.[33]

Botany and anatomy were closely intertwined in the sixteenth century. Both were increasingly studied by physicians in the sixteenth century, both relied on new ways of seeing and a new interest in direct personal observation, on printing to disseminate new concepts and technology, and, because both fields relied so heavily on visual studies, both also relied on new artistic realism for illustrations to accompany the textual information.[34] While demonstration dissections of cadavers had been practiced at many universities since the fourteenth century, the study of human anatomy gained new prominence through the combined efforts of anatomists and artists, particularly in Italy.[35]

Alchemy, botany, anatomy, and surgery were not just fields that embraced new forms of knowledge, they were fields that underwent drastic changes as a result of it. The new processes of experiment and firsthand observation were integral to the revival and expansion of these fields. Surgeons offer firsthand experiences throughout their texts, often after first citing ancient authorities then either challenging, amending, or adding their own perspective to the subject at hand. Juan Fragoso, discussing wounds infested with vermin (maggots), first refers to Paul of Aegina's teaching to remove the humid putrid matter. Then offering several recipes for compounds to apply to the wounds, he comments on a "great remedy" that he has "seen by experience in children's wounds."[36] Francisco Díaz, discussing symptoms of bladder stone, offers Avicenna's view of symptoms that indicate a large stone, then offers his own view that the symptoms are the same whether the stone is large or small, affirming, "[T]his I say from experience, that often I have seen this sign."[37] Such examples are extensive throughout all the sixteenth-century texts, offering individual experience and observation as legitimization for challenging or shifting knowledge.

At the same time, surgeons offered examples of specific patients they successfully treated to bolster the credibility and reliability of their innovations. Such use of case studies was not new, ancient and medieval surgical writers had also recounted stories of patients in their texts as they sought to codify the rational science of surgery.[38] They were, as Nancy Siraisi points out, in part a means of bridging theoretical and practical knowledge, showing successful application of theoretical knowledge.[39] Renaissance writers began to offer such case studies in new numbers and for new purposes. Gianna Pomata's study on the emergence of a new medical epistemic genre, known as *observationes*, shows the turn to observation, and the writing of case histories became widespread throughout medical culture in the later sixteenth century.[40] These texts were essentially compilations of case studies written by practicing physicians, offering a kind of testimonial to the authors' skill and success based on recounting actual practice rather than theory.

While the texts written by Spanish learned surgeons were not part of this genre, they also reflect the shift to emphasis on practice and practical application of theory.[41] Practicing physicians were already universally considered learned, so writing about practice was a useful way to demonstrate their abilities to apply theory. Practicing surgeons, in contrast, were acknowledged as skilled but not necessarily learned. In working to bridge the learned and practical traditions, surgeons demonstrated an ability to frame the physical problems they addressed with ancient authorities while offering these case studies as evidence of their skill in applying theory to practice. In discussing how to treat a subcutaneous bleed (ecchymosis) that occurs with a fracture but no open wound, Hidalgo de Agüero advises against lancing it open. He first gives his theoretical rationale for advising nonintervention, which centers on maintaining a concentration of natural heat necessary to heal the fracture and dissipate the excess blood. Opening the skin would dissipate body heat and allow ambient air to enter, potentially corrupting the interior. Hidalgo next examines several ancient authorities, including Celsus, Avicenna, and Hippocrates, who give differing opinions on the issue. Finally, he recounts his own work on a specific case when he was called to the town of Utrera to treat a man named Martin de Bohorques who had fallen from a horse and been knocked senseless for several days. Using only cupping glasses to lift the impressed cranial fracture and bandages, Hidalgo was able to see him to a full recovery in fourteen days. After recounting this case, he goes on to state, "[T]his question has been proved with reasons, authorities, and the experiences of great doctors who have tried one method and the other, coming cleanly to the truth" that less intervention is better.[42]

Juan Fragoso, in examining the complex question of when to remove a projectile that has caused a penetrating wound, not only references several contemporary surgeons but also recounts their case studies as exemplars. In a long passage that addresses the entwined issues of how accessible the object is, what it is made of, and what body parts (veins, arteries, organs) may be damaged or affected by its removal, Fragoso recounts specific cases described by other surgeons, including Pietro Argellata, Bartolomeo Maggi, Alonso Hierro, Francisco Arceo, and two unnamed surgeons.[43] The first of these, from Argellata, Fragoso uses to support his argument that a surgeon must be cautious about removing an arrow (or other object) that may have punctured a major vein or artery, as the object may be acting as a tamponade and removing it could prove fatal to the patient. The rest are all stories of patients with objects left in them (intentionally or unintentionally) that years later created abscesses and emerged or were removed from other parts of the body.

The specific case studies offered by surgeons not only show their application of theory (oftentimes to support new methods) but also serve as a reminder to us of the dangers of daily life in the early modern era. Hidalgo de Agüero's case described earlier resulted from falling off a horse being ridden for a festival, and such falls from horses or mules were common. Other cases he describes include a patient wounded by being kicked by a horse and another who was beaten by soldiers from a visiting galley ship. Francisco Arceo, in a discussion of treating head wounds in youths, describes several specific cases in which wounds were the result of a sword, a "blunt weapon launched from a crossbow," a mule kick, and an attack with a bronze candlestick.[44] One of Arceo's most memorable case studies of violent wounding comes in a discussion on treating facial wounds, where he recounts a patient who had been gored by a bull, the horn penetrating underneath his chin and extruding on the left cheek between the eye and nose. Arceo describes his approach to healing such a difficult wound, suturing the entry and exit holes, and treating the wound inside the mouth by repeated gentle washing with a compound of barley, rose, and pomegranate flower. The patient, he recounts, was successfully healed but left with a hole in his palate for which he improvised, devising a plug of cork wrapped in linen, which when inserted allowed him to speak, eat, and drink.[45] This particular patient Arceo leaves anonymous, which Andrés Oyola has suggested may have been because at the time the wound occurred, bullfights had been prohibited as religious celebrations in the aftermath of the Council of Trent. Perhaps Arceo felt the patient had paid a sufficient price for his participation and therefore provided him anonymity.[46] Certainly, though, if one wanted to verify the story, the patient would not be hard to identify. In most cases, Arceo and others not only recount general patient histories but also identify patients specifically, by name, by trade, and, often, by where they lived, making these cases tangible and offering verifiable witnesses.

The case studies offered by learned surgeons served various purposes. They demonstrated in specific terms their skills and success as practitioners, while also allowing surgeons to show the application of theory in a demonstration of learnedness. Surgeons relied upon and advertised their experiences as legitimation for innovation and to place themselves within a broader epistemic shift in medicine. Additionally, as shown in the next chapter, they used their experience to expand the range of issues treated by surgeons.

Refining Knowledge and Practice

Renaissance surgeons used their experiences to both refine and expand surgical expertise. Most of the surgical texts examined here were written late in the authors' careers, reflecting not a sudden moment of innovation but decades of practice and accumulated knowledge. The innovations offered in their texts can be roughly divided into three categories. First, they sought to refine existing knowledge and practice, exemplified by Bartolomé Hidalgo de Agüero's vía particular and Andrés Alcázar's refinement of the tools for trepanation and detailed discussion of neurosurgery. Second, many surgeons expanded the range of surgical expertise, exemplified by Francisco Díaz's treatise on urology, which pulled the field from the realm of the empiric to that of the learned surgeon, and Juan Fragoso's treatise on legal medicine or forensics, which helped establish surgeons as experts in reading signs of the body to determine cause of death and other legal questions. Third, surgeons worked to build new expertise for issues that ancient writers hadn't experienced, such as gunpowder wounds on the battlefield and new diseases including typhus and the Great Pox. This chapter examines the first of these categories, the refinement of existing knowledge, while the expansion of surgical expertise into new areas and their responses to entirely new challenges are discussed in the next chapter.

Refinements to the knowledge and practices of surgery were established within prevailing theory and rationales. Renaissance surgeons carefully framed their innovations within the existing intellectual system and offered a combination of learned theory and personal experience to justify their utility and acceptability. Nevertheless, many of these innovations faced debate and discussion. In Chapter 2, we saw one side of the interactions and connections among this community of surgeons, the mostly positive acknowledgment of one another's work. Here, we examine in greater detail the other side of their interactions, the disputes. These disputes are important for giving us an additional window into how knowledge was being constructed and tested.

Refining Wound Treatment

Among the most contentious refinements of practice, for Spanish surgeons at least, was general wound treatment. In the mid-thirteenth century, surgical texts began to discuss wounds as a category of surgical treatment rather than merely including wounds as part of anatomical discussions.[47] This became the surgeon's defining task, healing the ruptures of the body. Where divisions between physicians and surgeons existed, it was this—the physician treated the interior body, and surgeons healed the breaks and breaches to the exterior. In the phrase most commonly used from ancient times, the surgeon's task was to heal the *solutio continuitatis* or "solutions of continuity" (what for modern readers might be rendered more understandably as "dissolutions of continuity"). Surgeons had for centuries offered both techniques and theories for how to best handle wounds in the attempt to ensure healing—how much to intervene and how much to simply let nature and time have their way. As discussed previously, there were two methods of treating wounds, generally known as wet and dry healing, both of which could be traced to the ancients. What had come to be the standard approach was the wet method (called the *vía comun*, by Bartolomé Hidalgo de Agüero), which advocated keeping wounds covered and moist with various ointments to encourage the growth of new flesh. The formation of clean pus (*pus loable*, what in later times came to be known as "laudable pus") was seen as a positive sign of healing. This was distinguished from fetid pus, which was not a sign of healing and may have required further intervention in the placing of stents (cannulae) in wounds to drain them or applying medicines within them.[48] The alternate approach, commonly known as dry healing (called *vía particular* by Hidalgo de Agüero) was less interventional, advocating washing the wound with desiccants such as wine, barley water, or other distillations; pulling together the openings of the wound as best as possible; keeping the wound loosely covered without heavy ointments; and avoiding other interventions such as drainage tubes.

Wet and dry healing were not simple binary options for wound healing, however. Part of the difference in these approaches was the kind of wound to which they would be most beneficial. Galen's discussion of the two methods recounted at the beginning of the chapter was in response to a particular kind of head wound and after treatment by trepanning. As Michael McVaugh has pointed out, medieval rational surgeons recognized the difference between simple wounds, such as cuts or blade wounds, which would heal smoothly and easily with bandaging or perhaps some sutures to keep the skin together, and more complicated wounds that were larger and involved contusions or loss of flesh.[49] The more complex the wound, the more intervention was called for. But in practice, it seems that over time, for reasons not entirely clear, more intervention became the standard while the less-interventionist dry approach fell by the wayside. The dry method had been particularly advocated by several medieval surgeons from Ugo de Borgognoni (d. 1258) and his son Teodorico (d. 1296/8) to Henri de Mondeville (d. 1320), but by the fourteenth century, the wet method had won out, backed by Guy de Chauliac in his 1363 *Chirurgia magna*, a text often translated, copied, and later printed, making it highly influential. Thus, sixteenth-century surgeons who rejected traditional methods were in fact revisiting an old question. Hidalgo de Agüero acknowledges this but insists that although earlier authors set out the same principles of healing, "none perfected it as with divine grace it is now perfected…both with our greater experience and with the composition of the medicines we have developed."[50] By the sixteenth century, experience had become the key to refining technique.

Hidalgo de Agüero was not the only surgeon to reject constantly manipulating wounds, his colleague Francisco Arceo likewise advocated as little intervention as possible, especially when treating young patients. Recall Arceo's admonition to treat facial wounds with poultices (rather than stitches), a practice that Juan Fragoso disagreed with.[51] Arceo's text, written in Latin and published in Antwerp, raised no objections from his fellow Spanish surgeons, though it is clear many read him.[52] Hidalgo de Agüero, publishing a decade later in Castilian, by contrast, received tremendous opposition to nearly all parts of his advice on nonintervention. Why the great difference in reception? In large part, this was likely a result of the format in which he first published.

Hidalgo de Agüero had been head surgeon at the Hospital del Cardenal in Seville for decades when he published a small broadsheet outlining his approach to healing wounds (see Figure 3.1). In this very brief text, Hidalgo de Agüero did not explain his advice in any detail, but merely offered a very terse list of forty-nine statements regarding surgical treatment and anatomy. These "avisos" or admonitions read very similarly in some ways to Hippocrates's *Aphorisms*, which may have inspired Hidalgo de Agüero in the style of his composition. But where Hippocrates deals with diagnosis and prognosis of illness, Hidalgo de Agüero deals with treatment of specific physical disruptions. These terse statements could also be classified as theses, perhaps published for the purposes of debate. He covers the expected topics of wounds, fractures, and broken bones, nearly always advising using the least intervention possible, such as "[i]n penetrating chest wounds it is not necessary to use cannula of lead or silver, but all should be healed by closing them," and "a fractured arm or leg with a wound should be treated without a splint or cast." His advice also touches on issues of anatomy, most of which were points under some dispute within the medical community, such as "the human eye has only four muscles for movement," and "man does not have a *rete mirabile* and those who say otherwise are mistaken."

He also offers snippets of advice on treatment of eruptive diseases such as measles (*sarampion*), smallpox (*viruelas*), the Great Pox (*morbo gálico*), and erysipelas.[53]

The reaction to this initial small publication was immediate. Another surgeon in the city, Dr. Estrada, quickly denounced Hidalgo de Agüero's "dangerous" doctrine to the city council and demanded their intervention to stop him from teaching these ideas to others.[54] This initial debate was contained within Seville and the circle of practitioners there. While records of the initiation of this dispute (Estrada's charges and Hidalgo de Agüero's response and proposal for an empirical test of the two systems) are extant in the city council records, the outcome is not. However, Hidalgo de Agüero's continued work and his ultimate publication of a much larger text testify to his success in defending himself.

Two years later, a much larger and more public dispute erupted. Juan Fragoso, by then a prominent royal surgeon at the court in Madrid, issued a lengthy refutation to Hidalgo de Agüero's practices, this time as a printed treatise appended to his own substantial surgical text. The 1586 edition of Fragoso's *Cirugia universal* included four new treatises, including one entirely devoted to disputing the system of Hidalgo de Agüero, though Fragoso avoids naming him.[55] Fragoso, perhaps understandably, was alarmed by many of these pieces of advice, which not only contradicted standard theory and practice but also appeared with no explanations for them, no scholarly apparatus of reference to ancient theory, and no justification or support for why one should accept them. In turn, Hidalgo de Agüero addressed Fragoso's complaints in his later full treatise, *Tesoro de la verdadera cirugía y vía particular* (1604). Unlike Fragoso, Hidalgo de Agüero did not hesitate to name his opponent, entitling one treatise of his text, "Response of Doctor Hidalgo to Licenciate Fragoso."[56]

The printed dispute between Hidalgo and Fragoso offers an instructive window into not only surgical practices but also their views of empiricism and experience as a means of gaining and legitimizing knowledge. Fragoso and Hidalgo de Agüero were nearly exact contemporaries, both born around 1530 and both died in 1597. Equally interestingly, they most likely knew each other, or certainly knew *of* each other, as their professional lives overlapped for several years in Seville before Fragoso left to join the royal court in Madrid. Perhaps earlier personal interactions helped fuel their disputes, but no evidence of personal interactions between the two has come down to us.

Given that Fragoso wrote from Madrid and Hidalgo de Agüero from Seville, the debate between them could perhaps be framed in terms of center and periphery, the court versus the provinces. As the center of the Protomedicato and medical licensing, Madrid certainly held an intellectual priority of place. However, such a frame would unfairly place the court (and surgeons there) as strictly traditionalists, opposed to innovation. This was clearly not the case, as several of our innovative learned surgeons were also serving at court. Instead, Fragoso can be seen in both lights, as expanding the purview of surgeons by offering new kinds of texts and embracing new *materia medica*, while also defending many traditional practices. This debate, as with the others discussed in this chapter, must be seen instead as a conflict of individuals, their experiences, and their attempts to wrestle with when and how to challenge orthodoxy. Hidalgo de Agüero was arguing for empirical evidence, based not only on observation of individual cases but (importantly) also on the collective cases he had treated—a rudimentary compilation of survival rates was, for him, sufficient reason for rejecting tradition; Fragoso saw this new approach as dangerous and the evidence for it as insufficient.

Fragoso dismisses Hidalgo de Agüero's arguments by stating, "[T]he ancients previously cited have already experimented and found the safest and recommended [course of treatment]."[57] For Fragoso, if one is to accept the experience of another, the word of the ancients outweighed the word of one of his contemporaries. He felt no need to supplant their advice based on others' experiences, particularly when the advice offered came with no justifications for it. Significantly, Fragoso argues against the empiric (in the traditional definition), who may succeed in healing one case of head wound without intervention (that is, without trepanation) while a surgeon who does trepan may lose the patient in another. From this, the empiric will insist that his way is the only way in all cases, and had the surgeon not intervened, his patient would have lived. There is an echo here again of medieval surgical authors, such as Dino del Garbo, who in considering whether a skull fracture could be treated without intervention (elevation of a depressed bone, removal of bone fragments) asserted that empirics who only applied plasters to such wounds might get lucky and heal a patient occasionally, but the surer method was to follow ancient advice and intervene.[58] Given the lack of any explanatory apparatus in Hidalgo de Agüero's broadsheet, Fragoso assumed him to be using just such "empiric" reasoning—always applying plasters or medicines and never intervening. This, Fragoso argues, is exactly what is dangerous—to take one case or a few cases and use them to reject tradition. For while some head wounds may heal without intervention, others will not. Thus, for Fragoso, the collective experience of the ancients should be trusted more than just one person's (often somewhat limited) experience.

Juan Fragoso's balance of tradition and innovation leaned more toward tradition in this instance. He included in his *Cirugia universal* not only this treatise denouncing the innovations of Hidalgo de Agüero but also followed it with a treatise recounting the *Aphorisms* of Hippocrates in Latin with Castilian translation and explication. The *Aphorisms* was a foundation medical text, one which was translated and commented upon by numerous medical figures from Galen on, so there was no text more fitting for a traditionalist to include.[59] It was also a sign of his erudition and fluency in moving between Latin and Castilian, as well as his embrace of the vernacular. In turning to Hippocrates, Fragoso placed himself among the sixteenth-century medical humanists, reaching back to original Greek and Latin sources to supplement if not replace the more recent renditions of "Arabized" Galenism found in Avicenna (Ibn Sina) and others. His new Castilian translation and explanation of the *Aphorisms* show his strong belief in the legitimacy of his own knowledge and training and his interest in mediating this established knowledge to a new vernacular generation. In addition, given that the *Aphorisms* do not pertain to surgery, per se, but rather to diagnosis and prognosis of illnesses, Fragoso's inclusion of the *Aphorisms* further expanded the reach and expertise of surgeons beyond wounds to illnesses themselves. It may also have been an additional rejection of Hidalgo de Agüero's own list of surgical aphorisms, bringing attention back to the original ancient ones.

Fragoso's direct rejection of Hidalgo de Agüero's innovations rested in a wide range of sources, including not only classical ancients but also other contemporary learned surgeons, including Andrés Alcázar, Giovanni da Vigo, Jacopo Berengario da Carpi, and Gabriele Fallopio (the latter two best known for their anatomical studies). Fragoso can be seen, then, not as a conservative critic who rejected things simply because they were new or different, but as a thoughtful surgeon who kept abreast of new publications and evaluated each on what he believed to be their merits.

Hidalgo de Agüero, so roundly denounced in print by Fragoso, responded to the challenge by writing not only his larger compendium of surgery, complete with full scholarly apparatus of an explanatory preface, references to ancient sources, and his rudimentary statistics, but also an additional treatise specifically entitled "Response to the Propositions Offered by Licentiate Fragoso against the Advice Published by This Author in 1584."[60] Though he may have begun writing immediately, he did not complete the work until 1593, when it received approval for publication from royal authorities. It took another decade before it appeared in print, in part because of his own death in 1597. His son-in-law finally oversaw the publication in 1604, which means that Fragoso did not live to see it in print either. This larger work takes on the task of providing evidence for his propositions, in the form of experience, reason, and authority as shown in earlier examples in this chapter. The structure is that of a scholarly tome—a reprinting of his original list of precepts followed by first a one-page overview table of contents, then a detailed table of contents (which runs eight pages), and then an alphabetical listing of Latin and Greek terms with their definitions in Castilian, which are used in the work but might be unfamiliar to some readers. Hidalgo de Agüero uses these structures to frame the work as a learned and rational treatise which argues throughout nearly all 289 folios for his methods of healing in place of the standard approaches.

This debate over the proper approach to wound treatment did not end there, however. Both men had influenced (both directly as teachers/mentors and indirectly through their texts) numerous students and disciples. Both their works (still including the specific treatises against each other) continued to circulate in new editions. Fragoso's work was republished, often compiled with the work of others, including the urology of Francisco Díaz or the anatomy of Francisco Núñez, at least eleven times in the next century and several more times in the century after. Hidalgo de Agüero's text was republished twice, 1624 and 1654, but copies circulated widely into the New World. In addition, Hidalgo de Agüero had spent his career training students at the hospital, and several of them later published treatises of their own defending his system. Two years after Hidalgo's *Tesoro* appeared in print, his successor at the Hospital del Cardenal, Juan de Sosa Sotomayor, published a defense of the vía particular in his Latin surgical text.[61] The next year, Juan de Barrios, who held both Juan Fragoso and Juan Calvo as his mentors (having worked alongside both), included in his treatise, *Verdadera medicina, cirugía y astrología* (1607) a scathing denunciation of Hidalgo ("against doctor Hidalgo from Seville"), defending Fragoso's position on traditional surgical interventions. A decade later, another student of Hidalgo, Enrique Vaca de Alfaro, published a new comparison of the two systems, leaning toward the benefits of the vía particular but without entirely dismissing the tradition in the vía común. Instead, he advocates a sort of middle position.[62] Two additional supporters of Hidalgo's system published texts in the seventeenth century, Pedro López de Léon in 1628 and Pedro Gago de Vadilla in 1632.[63]

Revisiting and Refining Trepanation

Juan Fragoso began his attack on Hidalgo de Agüero with the example of trepanation, likely because the latter's broadsheet begins with a strong rejection of it in all cases: "in no cases of head wound should one trepan, nor lift bones." [64] Hidalgo de Agüero revisits cranial wounds in six of his subsequent statements, specifically warning against trepanation (using the terms *legrar*, *trepanar*, and *perforar el cráneo*) in four of them.[65] The practice had become an important point of discussion (and at times contention) among learned surgeons in the sixteenth century who were working to align textual knowledge and practice.

Ancient texts had advocated the benefits of manual intervention in many cranial traumas, including enlarging wounds to effectively remove bone splinters or foreign bodies, lifting depressed fractures, and opening holes in the cranium to relieve or prevent inflammation. But the technical difficulty of much of this and the potential problems were clear. By the later middle ages many surgeons, particularly empirics, seem to have avoided these interventions, instead using only plasters or medicaments to treat all head wounds. Dino del Garbo's reference to empirics who universally use only plasters for head wounds was explicit in arguing that doing so often resulted in the patient's death.[66] In the next century, Guy de Chauliac recounted the various approaches in his *Chirurgia magna*. He relates that some, such as Avicenna, Albucasis, and Guillermo da Saliceto, used interventions in all cases of head wounds, while others, including "some Paduans and almost all the French and English," rejected interventions using only "plasters and potions, good wine, and bandaging." That he cites no specific names for this practice is perhaps an indication again that this was used by unlettered empirics rather than scholarly surgeons who wrote treatises. Finally, he describes a middle ground, followed by some including Lanfranc of Milan, using potions in some cases of fresh wounds but trepanning or elevating bones in others after a period of days had passed. Guy de Chauliac supported this moderate approach, adding his own cautions, including avoiding already weakened patients and avoiding using the procedure during a full moon, which "augments and approximates the cranium on the third of the critical days."[67]

The tenuousness of head wounds and resultant hesitations of intervention in them is reflected in many other treatises as well. In the mid-sixteenth century, Pierre Haschaert warned of the dangers of "cheats, quacks and fast-talkers" who asserted that "everyone who is trephinated will die and that no-one should bring about a wound to the head."[68] Thus, in his promotion of complete nonintervention in cranial wounds in the *Avisos*, Hidalgo de Agüero appears again as unskilled, an empiric rather than a learned surgeon. But, as we have seen, his explication of these *Avisos* in his larger text reveals his full knowledge of Hippocrates, Galen, and other ancient and medieval authors. Like others of his era, he combined his book learning with his experiences to arrive at one position regarding head wounds: nonintervention. Taking a middle position was Francisco Arceo, who advocated a more cautious approach to deciding when to trepan. On the other side was Andrés Alcázar, one of the strongest advocates for intervention, whose experiences with and knowledge of neurosurgery were unmatched in Spain. Alcázar refined and expanded the surgeon's knowledge of how to treat cranial traumas by building on texts that had come before, adding in his own experiences and observations. In his 1573 treatise, *De recta curandorum vulnerum ratione et aliis ejus artis praeceptis libri II*, he provided a detailed discussion of the types of head wounds and their varying symptoms, along with his own changes and refinements to the tools of trepanation, which place him as one of the strongest advocates for manual interventions in head wounds (see Figure 4.1).

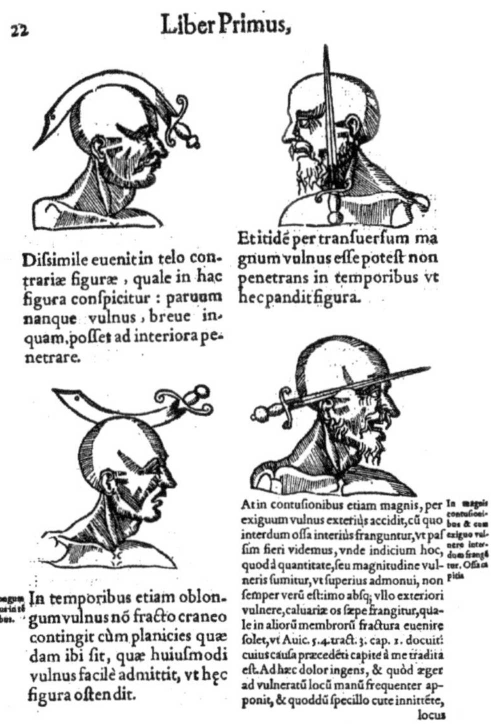

FIGURE 4.1 Illustration of head wounds from Andrés Alcázar, *Chirurgiae libri sex* (1575).

Detailed discussions of when and how to use trepanation were first expounded in the Hippocratic corpus, particularly in the treatise *On Head Wounds*, which advocated its use in many cases of both fractures and crush injuries.[69] The treatise sets out various approaches to opening the skull, including rasping (scraping) and using a trepan to drill through the skull (or nearly through, leaving a thin layer of bone to protect the membrane below). Among the pieces of practical advice offered, one which had a lasting influence was that of diagnosing the severity of a hidden fracture: expose the skull with a crossed incision to pull back the scalp (if needed) and rasp or scrape the cranium clean; next, rub a black substance onto it, allowing this to seep in before then washing and re-scraping the surface. The fracture will then show black against the newly whitened bone. One can determine the depth of a fracture by further rasping to determine if the black line disappears or remains embedded.[70] The treatise acknowledges several of the perils of trepanning, whether by scraping or drilling, cautioning the careful surgeon first that he not rupture or disturb the membrane (*dura mater*) under the skull, second that he place the trepan on the thickest bone possible, avoiding the sutures of the skull, and third that he frequently remove and cool the trepan in cold water to avoid overheating or scorching the bone.[71]

Later ancient medical writers, including Celsus and Galen, whose passage on the use of medicaments after trepanning opened this chapter, added details on the techniques of trepanning as well as descriptions of various instruments—the *terebra*, *modiolus*, and *abaptista*, as well as various knives, rasps, and forceps. Several of the Greek terms for the tools of trepanation were adapted first into Latin and later continued in use alongside other vernacular terminology. [72] The process of treating head wounds was recognized early on as a delicate one, which required different approaches depending on differing circumstances. This delicacy and complexity are reflected in the variety of tools developed for it as well as the adaptation and translation of the many terms used by surgeons. As shown by the earlier example of Hidalgo de Agüero, the vocabulary of both procedures and instruments grew increasingly complex over time. Berengario da Carpi, in his treatise on head wounds, *Tractatus de fractura calve sive cranei* (1518), commented on this profusion of terms for instruments and included illustrations of them to be as clear as possible.[73] In modern English usage, trephination and trepanation are used interchangeably, both terms based on names for the tool used—the trepan and the trephine. Sources agree that trepan is the older term, used by Greeks to describe the tool used to bore a hole in the skull. Trephine is believed to be a seventeenth-century term for a new type of tool with three points (tres fines), though scholars do not agree on who developed and/or popularized this.[74]

Terminology aside, there were many questions surrounding head wounds that continued to challenge Renaissance surgeons: which cases to intervene in, how much to intervene and with what instruments, and what medicaments to apply after or even instead. At the outset of the sixteenth century, Berengario da Carpi composed a treatise on head wounds, one of the first such to be printed. The *Tractatus de fractura calve sive cranei* (1518) was dedicated to Lorenzo de Medici, the

Duke of Urbino, who he had treated for a severe head wound by trepanning.[75] While da Carpi is perhaps better known as an early anatomist who was among the very earliest to reject pieces of ancient knowledge in favor of his own observations (such as the existence of the *rete mirabile*), his treatise on head wounds was also innovative and influential.[76] Da Carpi is among the many credited with innovations in the tools of trepanation, as well as laying out a clear explanation of when to use them. The treatise was certainly influential and referred to by many later learned surgeons, but it was not the last word, as surgeons throughout Europe continued to make their own observations and proffer their own opinions on head wounds based on experience.

The Duke of Urbino, wounded in battle, was not the first nor the last noble to suffer a serious head wound. Two additional famous cases of head injuries, those of King Henry II of France in 1559 and of Philip II's son and heir, Don Carlos in 1562, also reflect the ongoing debates over the use of trepanning. These two cases are connected not only in affecting royal families and by proximity in time but also by two of the attendants at each bedside, both of whom were employed by Philip II and recognized as outstanding members of their profession: Andreas Vesalius and Dionisio Daza Chacón. In both cases, these two were part of larger contingents of physicians and surgeons gathered to consult on treatment. Both cases reflect the uncertainty surrounding trepanation, as those in attendance debated the most effective regimens of treatment. While trepanation was dismissed as not useful in Henry II's case, it was initially attempted and then discarded for Don Carlos.

Henry II was wounded in the face and right eye by a shattered lance during a jousting tournament celebrating the Peace of Cateau-Cambrésis with Spain. As part of the peace, Philip II married Henry's daughter Elizabeth of Valois, though he did so by proxy, as he was otherwise occupied at the time in Brussels. Immediately upon Henry's wounding, a cadre of French royal physicians and surgeons were called to attend the king, including the chief physician Jean Chapelain and the royal surgeon Ambroise Paré. Dionisio Daza Chacón was in attendance, as he had accompanied Philip's proxy, the Duke of Alba, to Paris. While Daza Chacón later provided an important account of the events and treatment of the king, he is often forgotten in modern accounts. Even the detailed article by O'Malley and Saunders, which relies in part upon the account of Daza Chacón, neglects to mention his name or his presence among the doctors. He appears only in the footnotes.[77] Andreas Vesalius, who was at the height of his fame as an anatomist and surgeon, and also serving Philip II, was sent from Brussels, arriving a few days later. As a mark of his distinction, the collected medical men seem to have bowed to Vesalius as having leadership in this case, though he immediately pronounced the case hopeless.[78] While most modern accounts mention only the attendance of Paré and Vesalius, contemporary accounts refer repeatedly to a plurality of gathered physicians, though the others remain unnamed.[79] Henry II's case offers one of the more infamous instances of Renaissance use of experiment, as the Queen, Catherine de Medici, had four convicted criminals executed and donated their heads so that the doctors might attempt to replicate the wounding, dissect the heads and thereby determine the nature and extent of his interior injuries. This proved less useful than hoped, and ultimately after some debate, trepanation was rejected as useless in this case. Despite their collective best efforts, the king died after eleven days.[80]

Only a few years later, seventeen-year-old Don Carlos, only son and heir to Philip II, fell down a staircase and suffered a severe head injury.[81] He was living at the time in the city of Alcalá de Henares, as he suffered from quartan fevers (malaria) and the air there was considered healthier than that in Madrid.[82] Once again, Dionisio Daza Chacón was already on hand, as he was serving by then in the royal household as the prince's personal surgeon, alongside two royal physicians, Cristóbal de Vega and Santiago Diego Olivares.[83] These three were then joined by three additional physicians from Madrid, sent by Philip II upon hearing the news. When Carlos's condition took a turn for the worse, the group had to consider whether to trepan. As was common procedure, they chose first to enlarge the existing small wound in order to better examine the skull, debating what internal injuries might exist and whether opening the skull would be of help. Philip II then arrived from Madrid with two additional well-known doctors, Fernando de Mena and Andreas Vesalius. Thus, Daza Chacón and Vesalius were again reunited. Don Carlos's condition continued to deteriorate as the infection spread, and the eight doctors in attendance did not agree on whether to trepan. Vesalius was the strongest advocate in favor of it, a change from the earlier case. It was finally agreed to attempt it, as Don Carlos had become insensible. Even so, the initial scraping effort was quickly stopped when no cranial facture or damage was apparent, and it appeared Carlos's illness was a result of an external infection.[84] Further medical treatments were bolstered by religious efforts, which were ultimately credited by many for Carlos's eventual recovery.[85]

Both of these famous cases engendered debates among the attendant physicians. While many surgical treatises often seem to urge action over inaction for head wounds and to dismiss the use of plasters or ointments rather than intervention with knife and trepan, both of these cases were ultimately ones of inaction. None of the accounts left to us recall the specific arguments made or individual positions taken, but they tell us enough to be sure that there was ongoing debate among the medical men in attendance. In part, this reflected the delicacy of head wounds—each case needed to be considered individually, and there simply were no absolute rules to follow. In addition, the status of the patients certainly would have made all a bit more cautious in their approach. But the cases are stark reminders of the uncertainties that remained surrounding trepanation despite the increases in experience and improvements in tools.

Head wounds and the use of trepanation remained an aspect of surgical practice still under renovation throughout the sixteenth century. The questions surrounding diagnosing closed wounds or fractures and determining what invisible injuries might have resulted left room for experience and innovation. Dionisio Daza Chacón's attendance at two such famous cases of head wounds made him unusual, but all surgeons faced a variety of head injuries, and personal experience was likewise paramount for others writing about cranial trauma. Francisco Arceo, advocating for trepanation in cases of skull fracture without any obvious wound, recounts a case he had treated:

> During a brawl between two men, one hit the other in the head with a rock. The one that received the blow, despite wearing a helmet, fell immediately and when lifted by his friends he vomited. This vomiting along with a dent in the helmet made me think he had a hidden skull fracture which I confirmed when I located the site of the blow. The next day I trepanned his skull with the instrument known to Greeks as *abaptistón* and to us as trépano, …an abundance of black coagulated blood was expelled from the dura mater…the patient recovered without complications.[86]

Arceo uses this firsthand account to establish his experience and therefore authority on the topic, then goes on to discuss different types of trepans and how to use them. He advocated for trepanation in some cases but not all. For the most part, as discussed previously, he advocated for the least intervention in wounds possible, similar in many ways to Hidalgo de Agüero. He rejected outright, for example, the need to further open head wounds (or cutting open the skin if the initial blow had not done so), which had become standard among many surgeons as a means to ascertain the type and extent of injury. Such incisions, he pointed out, caused additional wounding that had to then be healed and prolonged the overall suffering of the patient. Instead, he advocated questioning the patient—what kind of object caused the wound? Did the patient fall to the ground? Did they lose consciousness? Arceo argues that such questions were a simpler method of evaluating the probability of any skull fracture and helped avoid unnecessary procedures.[87] Even those who accepted the need for such incisions sought to refine the practice. Though the ancient method was to cut an X or cross shape, some Renaissance surgeons began to advise a triangular one. Juan Fragoso disagreed with both, advising a simple lengthwise incision.[88] Arceo also rejected the need to trepan young people, advocating instead for the use of strong plasters to treat depressed fractures. Despite all these arguments, however, Arceo was a strong advocate of trepanning in certain cases and devotes several chapters of his text to a detailed discussion of it.[89]

Francisco Arceo's text, written in Latin, reached a wide European audience because it was first published in Antwerp and thereafter translated into various vernaculars through the late sixteenth and seventeenth centuries. Within Spain, however, it was Andrés Alcázar who was acknowledged as the preeminent authority on trepanation. Though he did not publish his text until late in his career, he had long been interested in trepanation, and as he recounts, he had worked early in his career to develop refinements to the standard tools then in use, creating "many tools never before seen or known to myself or my teachers" (see Figure 4.2).[90] According to Alcázar, his superior tools soon spread outside of Spain, first by Louis Delbourges, a royal surgeon who was attendant on Francis I while he was held captive by Charles V in Spain in 1525 and to whom Alcázar showed his work. Upon Delbourges's return to France the next year, he took with him these new

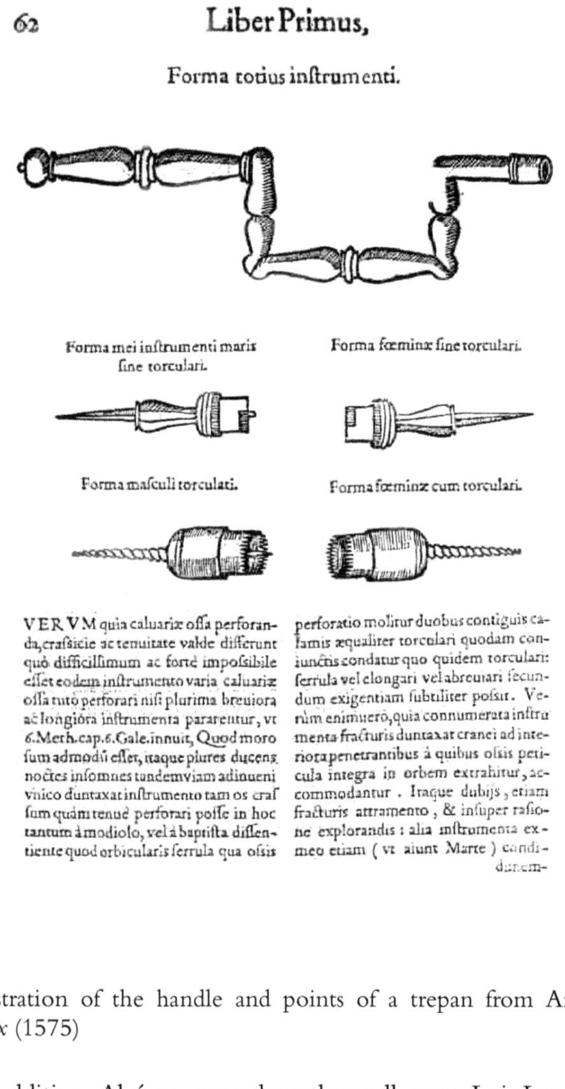

62 Liber Primus,

Forma totius inſtrumenti.

Forma mei inſtrumenti maris ſine torculari.

Forma fœminæ ſine torculari.

Forma maſculi torculati.

Forma fœminæ cum torculari.

VERVM quia caluariæ oſſa perforanda, craſsicie ac tenuitate valde differunt quò difficillimum ac fortè impoſsibile eſſet eodem inſtrumento varia caluariæ oſſa tutò perforari niſi plurima breuiora ac longiora inſtrumenta pararentur, vt 6. Meth. cap. 6. Gale. innuit, Quod moroſum admodũ eſſet, itaque plures ducens noctes inſomnes tandem viam adinueni vnico duntaxat inſtrumento tam os craſſum quàm tenue perforari poſſe in hoc tantum à modiolo, vel à baptiſta diſſentiente quod orbicularis ſerrula qua oſsis perforatio molitur duobus contiguis caſamis æqualiter torculari quodam coniunctis condatur quo quidem torculari ſerrula vel elongari vel abreuiari ſecundum exigentiam ſubtiliter poſsit. Verùm enimuero, quia connumerata inſtrumenta fracturis duntaxat cranei ad interiora penetrantibus à quibus oſsis pericula integra in orbem extrahitur, accommodantur. Itaque dubijs, etiam fracturis attramento, & inſuper raſione explorandis: alia inſtrumenta ex meo etiam (vt aiunt Marte) condidunem-

FIGURE 4.2 Illustration of the handle and points of a trepan from Andrés Alcázar, *Chirurgiae libri sex* (1575)

refinements. In addition, Alcázar accused another colleague, Luis Lucena, of taking these ideas with him when he left for what became several decades of study and travel in Italy and France. In later years, Alcázar accused the Italian Vidus Vidius (Guido Guidi) of usurping his ideas from Lucena and taking undue credit.[91] In fact, there is no shortage of sixteenth- and seventeenth-century figures credited with improvements to the trepanning tools or techniques, including Fabricius ab Aquapendente (Girolamo Fabrizio), Giovanni Andrea Della Croce, Berengario de Carpi, and John Woodall, another reflection of the wide range of practitioners engaged in Renaissance innovation.[92]

Whether or not we take Alcázar's claims of priority at face value, we can nonetheless credit him with an impressively thorough and advanced discussion of head trauma, neurological symptoms, and neurosurgery. Alcázar devoted the first book of his six-book work, *Chirurgiae libri sex*, specifically to cranial wounds and their effects on the peripheral nerves and nervous system. In these chapters, Alcázar remains grounded in ancient and medieval authors, such as Celsus, Galen, Avicenna, and Guy de Chauliac, but he continues to refer to his own experience or judgment using phrases such as "in my judgment" (*mio judicio*).[93] In describing symptoms of skull fracture, for example, he states, "It is a clear symptom of internal penetration when blood exits the fracture when the patient breathes shallowly or with difficulty. Nonetheless, it should be taken into account that blood flow from the fracture does not always indicate penetration" but only indicates it in certain circumstances. In summarizing the symptoms that may result from a blow to the head, he states that abscesses are possible, but "in my opinion rarely form immediately."[94] Though he does not offer colorful case studies, Alcázar's observations and experience permeate this treatise as he works to expand and refine the surgeon's understanding of head wounds.

Like the revised approach to wound healing advocated by Hidalgo de Agüero, Alcázar's advice on head wounds reflects the new interest of surgeons in refining existing knowledge and revising surgical approaches to significant issues. These two examples are a small reflection of the larger ongoing practices of new knowledge production among sixteenth-century surgeons. Indeed, the names of many such reforming surgeons appear in the texts and margins of all learned surgical texts: Giovanni da Vigo, Berengario da Carpi, Vidus Vidius, Gabrielle Fallopio, Ambroise Paré, Jean Tagault, and many more. In some cases, however, surgeons became innovators and reformers out of necessity as they faced new problems for which ancient authorities had no clear advice.

Notes

1 "Hallaras curioso lector en este tratado, todo el compenio de chyrurgia, dividido en quatro libros…La causa que me movio a publicar esta obrezilla, fue ver la falta que ay de libros, en que se pueden exercitar los Chyrurjanos romancistas…acorde imprimir, el presente tratado, y publicalle con sentencias y autoridades de gravissimos autores, ansi griegos como arabes…y no menos con la larga experiencia, que en muchos anos a que e trabajad, en muchos y muy insignes pueblos de Espana y principalmente en la ciudad de Burgos." Francisco Díaz, *Compendio de chirurgia: En el qual de trata de todas las cosas tocantes la theorica y pratica della* (Madrid, 1575), Prologo al lector.

2 Ian Maclean, *Logic, Signs and Nature in the Renaissance: The Case of Learned Medicine* (Cambridge University Press, 2007), 18–22.

3 Pamela H. Smith, Amy R. W. Meyers, and Harold J. Cook, eds., *Ways of Making and Knowing: The Material Culture of Empirical Knowledge* (Ann Arbor: University of Michigan Press, 2014); Sandra Cavallo, *Artisans of the Body in Early Modern Italy: Identities, Families and Masculinities* (New York: Manchester University Press, 2007).

4 "Y puedo afirmar como testigo de vista que e curado mas de veynte años, y tenido lugares publicos, como es el Hospital del Cardenal de Sevilla, y otros…è exercitado la particular por la misma orden por la comun, y è hallado tan grándes provechos que me han obligado, no solo a exercitarla, mas tambien a comunicarla." Bartolome Hidalgo de Agüero, *Tesoro de la verdadera cirugia y via particular contra la comun* (Sevilla, 1604), 32v.

5 "Y en los años que han curado mis antecessores, y yo por la comun, se halla mayor numero de los muertos que de los vivos." Hidalgo de Agüero, 32v.

6 Galen, *Method of Medicine* VI.6, ed. and trans. Ian Johnston and G. H. R. Horsley, The Loeb Classical Library 517 (Cambridge, MA: Harvard University Press, 2011), 233.
7 Allen G. Debus, *Man and Nature in the Renaissance*, Cambridge History of Science (Cambridge: Cambridge University Press, 1995), 19–33; Walter Pagel, *Paracelsus: An Introduction to Philosophical Medicine in the Era of the Renaissance* (New York: Karger Medical and Scientific Publishers, 1982).
8 Lilla Vekerdy, "Paracelsus's *Great Wound Surgery*," in *Textual Healing: Essays on Medieval and Early Modern Medicine*, ed. Elizabeth Lane Furdell (Boston: Brill, 2005), 89.
9 José Pardo-Tomás, "Autores médicos en los índices inquisitoriales españoles del siglo XVI," *Dynamis: Acta Hispanica Ad Medicinae Scientiarumque Historiam Illustrandam;* Vol.: 5–6 (1985); The appearance of Paracelsus in Spanish Indexes as of 1583 led to an early incorrect belief that he was unread and uninfluential in Spain. See José María López Piñero, "Paracelsus and His Work in 16th and 17th Century Spain," *Clio Medica* 8, no. 2 (1973): 113–41; More recent work has revised this view, particularly in relation to his alchemical studies. See Miguel López Pérez, "Spanish Paracelsus Revisited and Decontaminated," *Azogue* 7 (2010): 339–65. Nonetheless, Paracelsus's medical ideas seem to have had relatively small effect. While there were certainly proponents of chemical medicine, there was no distinct "paracelsian" movement.
10 Miguel López Pérez, "Spanish Paracelsus Revisited and Decontaminated," *Azogue* 7 (2010–2013): 352–3.
11 "[E]xpurgada conforme al nuevo catalogo, y expurgatorio del santo Oficio." Juan Fragoso and Francisco Díaz, *Cirugia vniuersal, aora nueuamenta añadida...: Iten otros quatro tratados, el primero es vna suma de proposiciones contra auisos de cirugia, el segundo de las declaraciones acerca de diuersas heridas y muertes, el tercero, de los Aphorismos de Hipocrates tocantes a cirugia, el cuarto, de la naturaleza y calidades de los medicamentos simples; Iten vn tratado de todas las enfermedades de los riñones, vexiga y carnosidades de la verga y orina y de su cura...; por Francisco Diaz...* (por la viuda de Alonso Martin, 1627), 514.
12 Vivian Nutton, *Ancient Medicine* (New York: Routledge, 2009), 147–50.
13 Susan P. Mattern, *The Prince of Medicine: Galen in the Roman Empire* (New York: Oxford University Press, 2013), 46–9.
14 Mattern, 48.
15 G. E. R. Lloyd, *The Revolutions of Wisdom* (Berkeley: University of California Press, 1989), 158–67; Susan P. Mattern, *The Prince of Medicine: Galen in the Roman Empire* (New York: Oxford University Press, 2013), 51–3; Jeremy Howick, "Aulus Cornelius Celsus and 'Empirical' and 'Dogmatic' Medicine," *Journal of the Royal Society of Medicine* 109, no. 11 (2016): 426–30, https://doi.org/10.1177/0141076816672397.
16 William Eamon, *The Professor of Secrets: Mystery, Medicine, and Alchemy in Renaissance Italy* (Washington, DC: National Geographic, 2010), 48, 243; Katharine Park, *Doctors and Medicine in Early Renaissance Florence* (Princeton, NJ: Princeton University Press, 1985), 66–7.
17 David Gentilcore, *Healers and Healing in Early Modern Italy*, Social and Cultural Values in Early Modern Europe (New York: St. Martin's Press, 1998), 109; William Eamon, *The Professor of Secrets: Mystery, Medicine, and Alchemy in Renaissance Italy* (Washington, DC: National Geographic, 2010), 40.
18 "[C]on cargo y obligación de curar piedras y roturas y otras cosas" Juan Manuel Jiménez Muñoz, *Médicos y cirujanos en "Quitaciones de Corte" (1435–1715)* (Valladolid: Universidad de Valladolid, 1977), 95–6.
19 Jiménez Muñoz, 23, 37; David C. Goodman, *Power and Penury: Government, Technology, and Science in Philip II's Spain* (New York: Cambridge University Press, 1988), 217–19.
20 Michele L Clouse, *Medicine, Government and Public Health in Philip II's Spain: Shared Interests, Competing Authorities*, 2011, 77; Gustav Ungerer, "George Baker: Translator of Aparicio de Zubia's Pamphlet on the 'Oleum Magistrale,'" *Medical History* 30, no. 02 (April 1986): 203–11; Rafael Muñoz Garrido, *Empiricos sanitarios españoles de los siglos XVI y XVII*, vol. 6, Cuadernos de Historia de La Medicina Española (Salamanca: Universidad de Salamanca, 1967).

21 "Como la experiencia sea madre de todas las cosas, y mas essencial que la teorica," Andres Leon, *Practico de morbo Gallico, en el quel se contiene el origen y conocimiento della enfermedad, y el mejor modo de curarla. Por el Doctor Andres Leon, … dirigido al Conde de Lemos, de quien el autor es vassallo, y criado*, (1605) Ch IIII, fol. 5.
22 Dionisio Daza Chacón, *Practica y teorica de cirugia en romance y en latin* (Valladolid: en casa de Ana Velez, 1609), 26–7; Juan Calvo, *Primera y segunda parte de la cirugia uniuersal y particular del cuerpo humano* (Madrid, 1674), 31–33; Bartolomé Hidalgo de Agüero, *Thesoro de la verdadera cirugía y vía particular contra la común* (Sevilla: Francisco Pérez, 1604), fols. 43–68.
23 Lawrence Principe, *The Secrets of Alchemy* (Chicago: University of Chicago Press, 2013).
24 Pamela H. Smith, *The Business of Alchemy: Science and Culture in the Holy Roman Empire* (Princeton, NJ: Princeton University Press, 1994); Tara E. Nummedal, *Alchemy and Authority in the Holy Roman Empire* (Chicago: University of Chicago Press, 2007); Karen Hunger Parshall, Michael Thomson Walton, and Bruce T. Moran, eds., *Bridging Traditions: Alchemy, Chemistry, and Paracelsian Practices in the Early Modern Era*, Early Modern Studies Series 15 (Kirksville, Missouri: Truman State University Press, 2015).
25 [25] William Eamon, *Science and the Secrets of Nature: Books of Secrets in Medieval and Early Modern Culture* (Princeton, N.J: Princeton University Press, 1994); Elaine Leong and Alisha Rankin, eds., *Secrets and Knowledge in Medicine and Science, 1500–1800* (Routledge, 2011).
26 Lawrence Principe, *The Secrets of Alchemy* (Chicago: University of Chicago Press, 2013).
27 Mar Rey Bueno and María Esther Alegre Pérez, "Los destiladores de Su Majestad. Destilación, espagiria y paracelsismo en la corte de Felipe II," *Dynamis: Acta Hispanica Ad Medicinae Scientiarumque Historiam Illustrandam* 21 (2001): 323–50; Francisco Javier Campos y Fernandez de Sevilla, ed., *La ciencia en el monasterio del Escorial* (Madrid: Ediciones Escurialenses, 1992).
28 Paula De Vos, "The Science of Spices: Empiricism and Economic Botany in the Early Spanish Empire," *Journal of World History* 17, no. 4 (2006): 399–427; Antonio Barrera-Osorio, *Experiencing Nature: The Spanish American Empire and the early Scientific Revolution*, (Austin, TX: University of Texas Press, 2006).
29 Josep L. Barona, "Clusius' exchange of botanical information with Spanish scholars" in *Carolus Clusius: Towards a Cultural History of a Renaissance Naturalist*, ed. Florike Egmond, Paul Hoftijzer and Robert P.W. Visser (Amsterdam: Koninklijke Nederlandse Akademie van Wetenschappen, 2007), 110.
30 Antonio Barrera-Osorio, *Experiencing Nature: The Spanish American Empire and the Early Scientific Revolution* (Austin, TX: University of Texas Press, 2006), 122–7; José Pardo Tomás, *Un lugar para la ciencia: escenarios de práctica científica en la sociedad hispana del siglo XVI* (La Orotava, Tenerife: Fundación Canaria Orotava de Historia de la Ciencia, 2006), 75–109.
31 Alix Cooper, *Inventing the Indigenous: Local Knowledge and Natural History in Early Modern Europe* (New York: Cambridge University Press, 2007); A. G. Morton, *History of Botanical Science: An Account of the Development of Botany from Ancient Times to the Present Day* (New York: Academic Press, 1981), 115–48.
32 Antonio Musa Brasavola, *Examen Omnium Simplicium* (1536), cited in A. G. Morton, *History of Botanical Science* (New York: Academic Press, 1981), p. 118.
33 The bibliography on early modern botany is quite extensive. A sampling of recent works would include Alix Cooper, *Inventing the Indigenous: Local Knowledge and Natural History in Early Modern Europe* (New York: Cambridge University Press, 2007); Florike Egmond, *The World of Carolus Clusius: Natural History in the Making, 1550–1610*, Perspectives in Economic and Social History, no. 6 (Brookfield, VT: Pickering & Chatto, 2010); Brent Elliott, "The World of the Renaissance Herbal," *Renaissance Studies* 25, no. 1 (2011): 24–41, https://doi.org/10.1111/j.1477-4658.2010.00706.x; Leah Knight, *Of Books and Botany in Early Modern England: Sixteenth-Century Plants and Print Culture*, (Burlington, VT: Ashgate, 2009); Sachiko Kusukawa, *Picturing the Book of Nature: Image, Text, and Argument in Sixteenth-Century Human Anatomy and Medical Botany* (Chicago: University of Chicago Press, 2012); Brian W. Ogilvie, *The Science of Describing: Natural History in Renaissance Europe* (Chicago: University of Chicago Press, 2006).

34 Kusukawa, *Picturing the Book of Nature.*
35 See introduction, note 2.
36 "Tiene se assi mismo por muy gran remedio (segun se ha visto por experiencia en llagas de niños)." Juan Fragoso, *Erotemas chirurgicos en los que se enseña todo lo mas necessario del arte de cyrurgia…* (por Pierres Cosin, a costa de Sebastian Yuañez, 1570), fol. 194.
37 "y esto hablo de experiencia, que muchs vezes he visto tener esta señal." Francisco Díaz, *Tratado, nuevamente impresso, de todas las enfermedades de los riñones, vexiga, y carnosidades de la verga y urina: dividido en tres libros* (Madrid, 1588), 207.
38 Cristina Álvarez Millán, "Graeco-Roman Case Histories and Their Influence on Medieval Islamic Clinical Accounts," *Social History of Medicine* 12, no. 1 (April 1, 1999): 19–43, https://doi.org/10.1093/shm/12.1.19; Cristina Álvarez Millán, "The Case History in Medieval Islamic Medical Literature: Tajārib and Mujarrabāt as Source," *Medical History* 54, no. 2 (April 2010): 195–214, https://doi.org/10.1017/S0025727300006712.
39 Nancy G. Siraisi, "How to Write a Latin Book on Surgery: Organizing Principles and Authorial Devices in Guglielmo Da Saliceto and Dino Del Garbo," in *Practical Medicine from Salerno to the Black Death*, ed. Luis García Ballester (New York: Cambridge University Press, 1994), 103.
40 Gianna Pomata, "Sharing Cases: The *Observationes* in Early Modern Medicine," *Early Science and Medicine* 15, no. 3 (April 1, 2010): 193–236.
41 These were also different from casebooks, such as those of Simon Forman and Richard Napier, which were not published. See Lauren Kassell, "Casebooks in Early Modern England: Medicine, Astrology, and Written Records," *Bulletin of the History of Medicine* 88, no. 4 (2014): 595–625.
42 "Assi de lo dicho queda nuestra question provada con razones, autoridades y experiencia de varones doctos que han exercitado lo uno y lo otro y han sacado en limpio esta verdad." Bartolomé Hidalgo de Agüero, *Thesoro de la verdadera cirugía y vía particular contra la común* (Sevilla: Francisco Pérez, 1604), 6v–7v.
43 Juan Fragoso, *Cirugia universal, aora nuevamente emendada, y añadida en esta sexta impression, por el licenciado Juan Fragoso médico, y cirujano del Rey nuestro señor, y de sus Altezas. Y mas otros quatro tratados. El primero es, una suma de proposiciones contra ciertos avisos de cirugia. El segundo, de las declaraciones acerca de diversas heridas, y muertes. El tercero, de los aforismos de Hippocrates tocantes a cirugia. El quarto, de la naturaleza, y calidades de los medicamentos simples* (Madrid: Viuda de Alonso Gómez, 1596), 142v–44.
44 Francisco Arceo de Fregenal, *Método verdadero de curar las heridas y otros preceptos de este arte: Método de curar las fiebres*, ed. Andrés Oyola Fabián and J. Cobos Bueno, Bibliotheca Montaniana 21 (Huelva: Universidad de Huelva, 2009), 136–9.
45 Francisco Arceo de Fregenal, *Método verdadero de curar las heridas y otros preceptos de este arte: Método de curar las fiebres*, ed. Andrés Oyola Fabián and J. Cobos Bueno, Bibliotheca Montaniana 21 (Huelva: Universidad de Huelva, 2009), 143.
46 Andres Oyola, "Cirugía Taurina en el siglo XVI," *Toros de Lidia* (blog), September 21, 2017, http://torosdelidia.es/cirugia-taurina-en-el-siglo-xvi/.
47 Michael R. McVaugh, *The Rational Surgery of the Middle Ages*, Micrologus' Library 15 (Firenze: SISMEL, Ed. del Galluzzo, 2006), 91–2.
48 McVaugh, 103–6; Nancy G. Siraisi, *Medieval & Early Renaissance Medicine: An Introduction to Knowledge and Practice* (Chicago: University of Chicago Press, 1990), 169–70.
49 McVaugh, *The Rational Surgery of the Middle Ages*, 94–5.
50 "Y assi concluyo que aunque estos autores graves dieron principio a esta via, nunca la perficionaron, como por la divina gracia en nuestros tiempos esta perfeta…asi con nuestra larga experiencia como con la composicion de las medicinas que para este efecto hemos inventado." Hidalgo de Agüero, *Thesoro de la verdadera cirugía y vía particular contra la común*, fol. 81v.
51 Chapter 2, note 70.
52 José Miguel Cobos and José Ramón Vallejo, "Francisco Arceo, médico del Santo Oficio de la Inquisición de Llerena," *Inquisición: XV Jornadas de historia en Llerena*, 2014, 301; José López Piñero et al., *Diccionario Histórico de La Ciencia Moderna En España*, 1a ed., vol. I (A–L) (Barcelona: Península, 1983), 64.

53 Hidalgo de Agüero, *Thesoro de la verdadera cirugía y vía particular contra la común*. The *avisos* are reprinted as front matter in his published text. The examples cited are statements 16, 24, 32, 33, 25, and 44. For discussion of the debate on the *rete mirabile*, see John M. Forrester, "The Marvellous Network and the History of Enquiry into Its Function," *Journal of the History of Medicine and Allied Sciences* 57 (2002): 198–217.
54 Esteban Torre, "Las 'conclusiones' del doctor Estrada de Madrid, contra los 'Avisos Particulares' del doctor Hidalgo de Aguero, Sevillano," *Asclepio* 30/31 (79 1978): 389–401; Kristy Wilson Bowers, "Tradition and Innovation in Spanish Medicine: Bartolomé Hidalgo de Agüero and the Vía Particular," *Sixteenth Century Journal* XLI, no. I (2010): 29–47.
55 Juan Fragoso, *Cirugia universal, aora nuevamente emendada, y añadida* (Madrid: Viuda de Alonso Gómez, 1586). The treatise in question is titled "Suma de las proposiciones de cirugia, que el licenciado Fragoso enseña contra unos avisos que imprimió un Doctor desta facultad, el año de mil y quinientos y ochenta y quatro."
56 "Respuesta de el Doctor Hidalgo al Licenciado Fragoso" Bartolome Hidalgo de Aguero, *Tesoro de la verdadera cirugia y via particular contra la comun* (Sevilla, 1604), fols. 144–93.
57 "los Médicos mas antiguos que alega ya tendrian experimentado, que lo mas seguro, y que convenia." Fragoso and Díaz, *Cirugia uniuersal, aora nueuamenta añadida…*, 516.
58 Nancy G. Siraisi, "How to Write a Latin Book on Surgery: Organizing Principles and Authorial Devices in Guglielmo Da Saliceto and Dino Del Garbo," in *Practical Medicine from Salerno to the Black Death*, ed. Luis García Ballester (New York: Cambridge University Press, 1994), 60–1.
59 Antònia Carré, "The Medieval Catalan Translations of Hippocrates' 'Aphorisms'," trans. Andrew Stacey, *Sciència.cat: La ciència en la cultura catalana a l'Edat Mitjana i el Renaixement*, September 29, 2017, https://sciencia.cat/temes/medieval-catalan-translations-hippocrates-aphorisms.
60 *Respuesta a las proposiciones que el Licenciado Fragoso enseña, contra unos avisos particulares de Cirugia que imprimio el Autor, Ano 1584.*
61 Joaquín Herrera Dávila and José Joaquín Jadraque Sánchez, "El 'Tractatus de curatione' – 1606 – de Juan Sosa Sotomayor," *Archivo hispalense: Revista histórica, literaria y artística* 91, no. 276 (2008): 93–129.
62 Enrique Vaca de Alfaro, *Proposicion chirurgica i censura iudiciosa entre las dos vias curativas de heridas de cabeça comun i particular i elecion desta: con dos epistolas al fin, una de la naturaleza del tumor preternatural, i otra de la patria i origen de Auicena…* (Sevilla: por Gabriel Ramos Vejarano, 1618).
63 Pedro López de León, *Pratica y teorica de las apostemas en gneral y particular: Questiones y praticas de cirugia de heridas, llagas y otras cosas nuevas y particulares* (Sevilla: en la Oficina de Luys Estupiñan, 1628); Pedro Gago de Vadilla, *Discursos de verdadera cirugia, y censura de ambas vias, y eleccion de la primera intencion curativa y unicion de las heridas* (Madrid, 1632) Both of these texts were also reprinted several times over the century. See also Jairo Solano Alonso, *Salud, cultura y sociedad: Cartagena de Índias, siglos XVI y XVII* (Barranquilla: Universidad del Atlántico, 1998).
64 "que en ninguna herida de cabeza se a de legrar, ni levantar huessos" Hidalgo de Agüero, *Thesoro de la verdadera cirugía y vía particular contra la común*, 2v.
65 Avisos 1, 4, 5, 6, 13 all warn specifically against trepanation, while 12 and 14 refer to head wounds without specific mention of it.
66 Nancy G. Siraisi, "How to Write a Latin Book on Surgery: Organizing Principles and Authorial Devices in Guglielmo Da Saliceto and Dino Del Garbo," in *Practical Medicine from Salerno to the Black Death*, ed. Luis García Ballester (New York: Cambridge University Press, 1994), 60–1.
67 W. A. Brennan, trans., *Guy de Chauliac (A.D. 1363) on Wounds and Fractures* (Chicago: W.A. Brennan, 1923), 83–4.
68 Robert Van Hee, "The Evolution of Surgery in the Low Countries during the Sixteenth Century," *Sartoniana / University of Ghent Sarton Chair of the History of Sciences* 15 (2002): 115.

69 Hippocrates, *On Head Wounds*, trans. Maury Hanson, vol. I 4,1, Corpus Médicorum Graecorum (Berlin: Akademie Verlag, 1999), 9.2.
70 Hippocrates, *On Head Wounds*, 14.2–8.
71 Hippocrates, *On Head Wounds*, 12.4, 21.1–3.
72 See, for example, the discussion in José M González-Darder, *Trepanation, Trephining and Craniotomy: History and Stories* (Springer Nature, 2019), 9–16; Charles G. Gross, *A Hole in the Head: More Tales in the History of Neuroscience* (Cambridge, MA: MIT Press, 2009), 8–10. In modern English, trepan and trephine (a seventeenth-century term) are often used interchangeably as both noun and verb to refer to both the process and the specific instrument used, though trephine has become the more common. Modern neurosurgeons use a variety of more specific terms to distinguish, for example, small openings (burr holes) from larger ones (cranial flaps).
73 L. R. Lind and Berengario da Carpi, "Berengario Da Carpi on Fracture of the Skull or Cranium," *Transactions of the American Philosophical Society* 80, no. 4 (1990): 134–5, https://doi.org/10.2307/1006547.
74 José M González-Darder, *Trepanation, Trephining and Craniotomy: History and Stories* (Springer Nature, 2019), 13–14, https://doi.org/10.1007/978-3-030-22212-3.
75 L. R. Lind and Berengario da Carpi, "Berengario Da Carpi on Fracture of the Skull or Cranium," *Transactions of the American Philosophical Society* 80, no. 4 (1990): xii, https://doi.org/10.2307/1006547.
76 John M. Forrester, "The Marvellous Network and the History of Enquiry into Its Function," *Journal of the History of Medicine and Allied Sciences* 57, no. 2 (2002): 206.
77 Charles Donald O'Malley and J. B. de C. M. Saunders, "The 'Relation' of Andreas Vesalius on the Death of Henry II of France," *Journal of the History of Medicine and Allied Sciences* 3 (1948): 197–213.
78 Charles Donald O'Malley and J. B. de C. M. Saunders, "The 'Relation' of Andreas Vesalius on the Death of Henry II of France," *Journal of the History of Medicine and Allied Sciences* 3 (1948): 206. This article also contains the text of Vesalius's postmortem examination of Henry II.
79 Dionisio Daza Chacón, "Relación verdadera de la herida de cabeza del Serenísimo Príncipe D. Carlos Nuestro Señor, de gloriosa memoria, la cual se acabó en fin de Julio del año de 1562," *Colección de documentos inéditos para la historia de España.* XVIII (1851): 537–63; Lucien Romier, *Les origines politiques des guerres de religion* (Paris: Perrin, 1913), 381–2; Charles Donald O'Malley and J. B. de C. M. Saunders, "The 'Relation' of Andreas Vesalius on the Death of Henry II of France," *Journal of the History of Medicine and Allied Sciences* 3 (1948): 204.
80 There are several accounts of Henry's accident and treatment. Though outdated in several ways (for example, describing Henry II's wife, Catherine de Medici, as "crafty and unscrupulous"), O'Malley and Saunders offer an excellent survey of the primary sources. Charles Donald O'Malley and J. B. de C. M. Saunders, "The 'Relation' of Andreas Vesalius on the Death of Henry II of France," *Journal of the History of Medicine and Allied Sciences* 3 (1948): 197–213.
81 There are several firsthand accounts of this case, notably that of Dionisio Daza Chacón, (see note 79); See also L. J. Andrew Villalon, "Putting Don Carlos Together Again: Treatment of a Head Injury in Sixteenth- Century Spain," *Sixteenth Century Journal* 26, no. 2 (1995): 347–65.
82 Andrew Villalon, "The 1562 Head Injury of Don Carlos: A Conflict of Medicine and Religion in Sixteenth-Century Spain," *Mediterranean Studies* 22, no. 2 (2014): 97.
83 Dionisio Daza Chacón, "Relación verdadera de la herida de cabeza," 538.
84 Villalon, 100.
85 Villalon, 95–134.
86 José María López Piñero, *La trepanación en España; clásicos neuroquirúrgicos españoles* (Madrid: Editorial Técnica Española, 1967), 100.
87 Arceo de Fregenal, *Método verdadero de curar las heridas y otros preceptos de este arte*, 116–17.

88 Fragoso and Díaz, *Cirugia uniuersal, aora nueuamenta añadida*..., 312.
89 José María López Piñero, *La trepanación en España; clásicos neuroquirúrgicos españoles* (Madrid: Editorial Técnica Española, 1967), 83, 99–103.
90 Andrés Alcázar, *Chirurgiae libri sex: in quibus multa antiquorum, et recentiorum sub obscura loca hactenus non declarata interpretantur* (Salamanca, 1575), 60.
91 Antonio Herrera Casado, "Andrés Alcázar, Cirujano Del Renacimiento," in *Gran Enciclopedia de Castilla-La Mancha*, vol. I (Zaragoza: Unión Aragonesa del Libro, 1982), 115.
92 José M. González-Darder, *Trepanation, Trephining and Craniotomy: History and Stories* (Springer Nature, 2019), 13, 131–86; Antonio Di Ieva et al., "Berengario Da Carpi: A Pioneer in Neurotraumatology: Historical Vignette," *Journal of Neurosurgery* 114, no. 5 (May 1, 2011): 1461–70.
93 Andrés Alcázar, *Chirurgiae libri sex*, 23.
94 José María López Piñero, *La trepanación en España; clásicos neuroquirúrgicos españoles* (Madrid: Editorial Técnica Española, 1967), 114.

5

EXPANDING SURGICAL EXPERTISE

Addressing New Problems

Andrés de León begins his 1605 surgical treatise with anatomy, an increasingly common subject for surgeons to include. His second book, however, shifts away from the practical knowledge of the body to a philosophical discussion of the rational soul (*anima*) by which God has distinguished man from lower animals. In this lengthy section (ninety folios divided into 153 chapters), León offers a Galenic definition of the art of medicine; a lengthy discussion of the importance of understanding astrology and the zodiac for prognostication (which includes several astrological charts); definitions of humoral theory, which includes elements, humors, temperaments, faculties; causes and signs of different fevers; and how to use pulse and urine diagnostically. All of these topics incorporated a great deal of theory about the body and its functioning. While most surgeons do not address nearly this much theory, others, including Juan Calvo, Dionisio Daza Chacón, and Bartolomé Hidalgo de Agüero, do offer definitions of medicine (as both art and science), discussing the role of humors and temperaments in causing illness, the effectiveness of particular treatments, and the theory of naturals, non-naturals, and contra-naturals. León also spends several pages defining both "art" and "science" in philosophical terms, stating, for example, "The arts, according to Aristotle, are of three types, some called contemplative, some active, and others effective, which are distinguished by reason of their objectives."[1]

Closely related to the refinements or innovations of treatment offered by learned surgeons was the expansion of surgical expertise into new areas of practice. This expansion is visible in their texts, where surgeons included new topics and redefined the domain of surgery within medicine. Ancient writers had supplied a tripartite definition of medicine: diet or regime, medicaments, and surgery. Learned surgeons blended the latter two categories together. They now defined surgery as both art and science, encompassing theory and practice.[2]

DOI: 10.4324/9781003291060-6

Literate surgeons in the thirteenth and fourteenth centuries had incorporated an increasing number of conditions in their texts, adding discussions of apostemes, cataracts, hernia, bladder stones, scabies, and other new skin diseases.[3] This was in part the result of the ongoing translation and circulation of Arabic texts, which offered a new theory for the causes of these conditions as well as their treatment. Over the intervening centuries, several of the previously mentioned conditions (cataracts, hernia, bladder stones) had increasingly been relegated to empirics or specialists. Renaissance learned surgeons once again paralleled the medieval tradition by widening the scope of a surgeon's expertise. This expansion of expertise is where we can most easily find the blurring of boundaries between physicians, surgeons, and empirics. Learned surgeons now included in their texts information on how to treat broken bones, dental problems, and bladder stones, all things that in recent times had been left to the treatment of empirics. They also included aspects of medicine that combined the theoretical with observational, such as forensic medicine, theories of disease, and antidotaries that offered instructions on how to make and apply a wide range of compound medicines. Indeed, some wrote specifically about medicine and surgery as distinct subjects, such as Juan Calvo's *Libro muy util y provechoso de medicina y cirugía* (1591) and Andrés de León's *Tratados de medicina, cirugía y anatomía* (1605). As part of shifting the boundaries of what surgeons were qualified to treat, many learned surgeons wrote about entirely new problems. The most well-known of these was gunpowder wounds resulting from the increased use of this relatively new weaponry on the battlefield, but we will also include in this category the understanding, diagnosis, and treatment of "new" epidemic diseases, including typhus and the Great Pox (morbo gálico), both of which were identified as new by Europeans in the 1490s. The causes of, nature, and effective treatments for these new diseases, along with the older disease plague, continued to be debated by both physicians and surgeons throughout the sixteenth century and beyond.

If we think of surgeons, particularly learned surgeons, as situated in the middle of a spectrum that ran from physicians down to empirics, we can see learned surgeons stretching outward from the middle, through those imaginary boundaries both below and above them, embracing and offering their own empiric practices while also encoding those practices in theory and textual knowledge. Here, we will examine various examples of how surgeons incorporated new knowledge in their texts, expanding the range of surgical expertise.

Urology

While urinary infections, bladder and kidney stones, and other urogenital problems were extremely common in the premodern world, for centuries they were generally treated by empirics or specialists. Of the many empirics employed by Philip II, specialists in treating urological disorders were the most common. While many surgical texts discussed various issues of the kidneys and bladder, they did so only in small pieces. Some include the kidneys and bladder in anatomical discussions, while others discuss treatment of penetrating abdominal wounds that affected them.

Some offer remedies, for example, for blood in the urine, while others mention suppression of the urine or inability to urinate.[4] This issue of blockage or stricture of the urethra, known in Spanish as "carnosidades de la vía de la urina" was one problem increasingly addressed in many surgical texts as a new method of treatment was spreading across Europe in the sixteenth century.

Francisco Díaz's 1588 text, *Tratado nuevamente impresso, de todas las enfermedades de los riñones, vexiga, y carnosidades de la verga, y urina* [New Treatise on All Conditions of the Kidneys, Bladder and Urinary Blockages] helped establish urology as a field of surgical expertise, overseen by learned surgeons who could diagnose and treat all manner of problems with the bladder, kidneys, and urinary tract (Figure 5.1). Díaz points out the piecemeal nature of current work, noting that "although the highly esteemed Spanish doctor [Andrés] Laguna and Doctor Romano wrote on urinary blockages…it was very brief and barely allowed one to understand what this problem was. And if Galen and other respected authors wrote on ailments of the kidneys and bladder, it was sprinkled about in various treatises and not gathered into one place."[5] Díaz not only collected pieces of this knowledge from diverse authors in multiple treatises, but he also systematized and then refined it, essentially creating a new medical field.

Collecting and codifying this piecemeal knowledge, Díaz then utilized his own expertise to refine the techniques and craft new instruments for the procedures he advocated. Díaz was well positioned to give this formerly practical topic new intellectual weight and legitimacy. By the time he compiled his text, Díaz was a well-established practitioner and scholar who had served as a royal surgeon for nearly two decades. He had extensive university training, earning multiple degrees. He was also known as a poet, whose friendship with other writers resulted in Miguel de Cervantes including him by name in *La Galatea* (1585) and Lope de Vega composing two sonnets for his urological treatise. Díaz was thus able to utilize his standing at court and among men of letters to give urology new legitimacy as a medical specialty that deserved detailed attention from qualified surgeons.

The dedication, prologue, and first chapter of Díaz's manual all address why this text needed to be written, a reflection, perhaps, that Díaz anticipated potential pushback for various reasons. Díaz seems to be addressing the potential controversy for offering an open discussion of difficult private problems as well as for bringing empiric or unlearned practices into a learned framework. He begins with an address to the Protomédico and personal physician to Philip II, Francisco Valles. He explains the need for and utility of his text, positioning himself as mediating ancient knowledge and modern practices, revealing "secrets" so that all may benefit. Books revealing the "secrets of nature," which included such things as medicinal, alchemical, and cosmetic recipes, were common in the mid-sixteenth century.[6] But while most of those books purported to take ancient and arcane knowledge and reveal it in modern understandable terms for the common man, Díaz was instead interweaving ancient theory and specialized knowledge of the practiced empiric. Though he wrote in the vernacular, his audience was practicing surgeons, and his stated purpose was to improve their practices. He refers specifically to Andres Laguna, the

TRATADO
NVEVAMENTE
IMPRESSO, DE TODAS
LAS ENFERMEDADES DELOS
Riñones, Vexiga, y Carnoſidades dela verga, y Vrina, diuidido en tres libros. Compueſto por Franciſco Diaz Dotor en Medicina, y maeſtro en Filoſofia, por la inſigne vniuerſidad de Alcala de Henares, y Cirujano del Rey nueſtro Señor.

DIRIGIDO AL DOTOR VALLE
Protomedico del Rey nueſtro Señor, y Medico

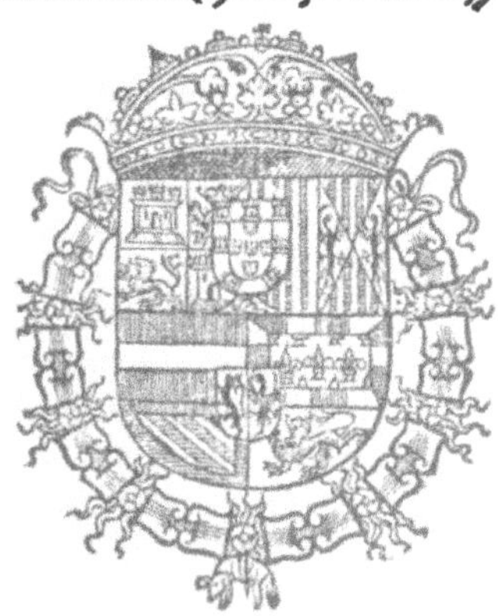

CON PRIVILEGIO.
Impreſſo en Madrid por Franciſco Sanchez.
Año. 1588.

FIGURE 5.1 Title page from Francisco Díaz, *Tratado nuevamente impresso de todas las enfermedades de los riñones, vexiga, y carnosidades de la verga, y urina* (1588).

highly learned physician who had passed away thirty years earlier, but whose work remained preeminent among Spaniards, and to Dr. Romano (Alfonso Díaz, no relation), the Italian who was more empiric than learned doctor but whose method of treating urinary blockages had grown popular across Spain and which Díaz himself used and promoted. With these two figures, Díaz lays out the parameters of modern knowledge—learned and empiric, textual and practical.

The initial dedication address is followed by a prologue to the reader in which Díaz makes another appeal to the value of modern or current knowledge, using as an example the relative ease with which morbo gálico was being cured in his time, as compared to the previous century when it was first recognized. Likewise, he argues, this urological information he was divulging was useful, important, and newly refined through his experience. And though he anticipated "no shortage of grumblers or backbiters," he urged the reader to overlook anything they felt should not be discussed (brought to light), and they would find much that was useful.[7] Finally, the first chapter of the text itself is entitled "In which is treated the motivations of this author to write of these ailments." Here Díaz again justifies the propriety of the subject matter as one also discussed at least in passing by many ancient authors, as well as one which he has had long experience in treating.

The most notable piece of empiric practice discussed by Díaz was a new method of removing urinary blockages not caused by stones. He embraced (and justified his embrace of) empiric practice by recounting the lack of information in ancient texts. He was certain, he states, that ancients must have named this ailment and discussed its remedy. Despite his great diligence in searching many authors, however, he did not find sufficient discussion of it anywhere. Nor did the Arabs seem to have much to say either. While both Galen and Avicenna do mention suppression of urine, neither (according to Díaz) explains it sufficiently or has much discussion of its causes or cure. Moving on to his own time, Díaz sets about giving credit where it was due. According to his account, an effective treatment was developed only in the early sixteenth century by a virtually unknown figure, a surgeon who Díaz names as "master Philip" who worked for Emperor Charles V in the Holy Roman Empire. Charles suffered from such stricture and master Philip successfully used a tube coated in caustics threaded up into the urethra to clear out fleshy growth and open the blockage. His success in treating the emperor led to other high-profile patients, including the Admiral of Naples. His successful method was learned by a young Roman pharmacist who worked with him and who then took this method back to Rome, gaining great fame and success for his use of it. In turn, this unnamed pharmacist trained a young Portuguese apprentice named Alfonso Díaz who brought the treatment to Spain in the 1550s, becoming known as Dr. Romano. Romano's success in treating members of the court while in Valladolid led Philip II to offer him a royal salary, charging him with not only curing those in the city in need of his services but also with teaching his techniques to all who wished to learn.[8] Thus Díaz himself came to learn and practice this same treatment and to improve upon it by developing new catheters and the use of different caustics (Figure 5.2). After recounting this early history, his treatise goes on for another eleven chapters carefully laying out the definitions, causes, and best treatment of these "carnosidades."

The treatise on urinary strictures was the third and last part of Díaz's larger treatise on urology, the first two parts of which examined the problems, causes, and treatments for ailments of the kidneys and bladder, respectively. The text as a whole was a revolutionary work that brought into a cohesive discussion all the potential urological conditions and established the surgeon, rather than the empiric, as the

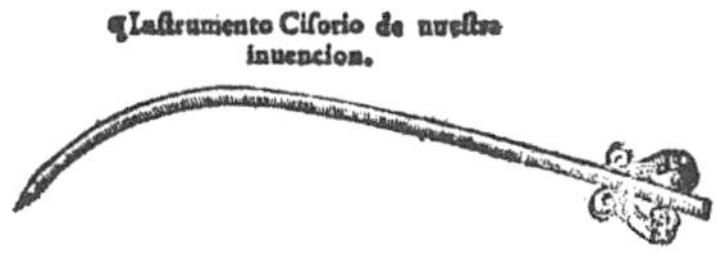

FIGURE 5.2 Illustration of a tool developed by Francisco Díaz to treat urethral stricture. Francisco Díaz, *Tratado nuevamente impresso de todas las enfermedades de los riñones, vexiga, y carnosidades de la verga, y urina* (1588).

best figure to offer diagnosis and treatment. Following Díaz's text, other physicians and surgeons also published on urinary problems, such as Francisco Sánchez de Oropesa, a physician in Seville, whose 1594 treatise was written specifically for a friend, Diego Enriquez León.[9]

Legal and Forensic Medicine

"In 1588, here in Madrid, a man having words with a woman suddenly died and the judge gathered a number of surgeons to determine the cause of death."[10] This case was recounted by Juan Fragoso in a brief treatise added to his *Cirugía universal*, entitled, "On the pronouncements surgeons have to make, regarding various conditions and many causes of death that may occur."[11] The reliance of courts on medical expertise was not new in the sixteenth century. Testimonies from a range of medical practitioners, particularly on matters relating to cause of death, had long been sought and offered in courts throughout continental Europe from the thirteenth century on.[12] In the Iberian Peninsula, the late thirteenth to early fourteenth centuries saw the emergence of a specific term for the medical expert witness, the *desospechador* (in Castilian) or *dessospitador* (in Catalan), who could give testimony on the causes and likely outcome of wounds, as well as causes of death and other legal matters.[13]

What emerged in the sixteenth century was an effort to codify in texts the range of legal issues that fell within the purview of medical expertise and guidelines on how to determine these issues. The questions surrounding causes of death were diverse: determining the cause of sudden or mysterious deaths, such as the circumstances quoted earlier; determining the lethality of wounds, signs of death from unusual causes such as lightning strikes, envenomation, and infanticide; detecting if overt signs of death such as hanging, drowning, or wounding were actually inflicted on the body after death; how to determine if a body that appears dead was, in fact, still alive. The other large preoccupation of these texts was legal questions related to sexuality and procreation, such as determining virginity, sterility, impotence, the possible length of pregnancy (which could speak to the legitimacy of the child), and so forth.

The most extensive and influential early modern text on legal medicine was *Quaestiones médico-legales* (1621–61) by the Italian physician Paulo Zacchia (1584–1659). Prior to this, however, there were many sixteenth-century authors who broached the topic to varying extents, each of whom has been credited at various times as the "founder" of forensic medicine. These included Ambroise Paré (*Traité des rapports*, 1575), Giovanni Filippo Ingrassia (*Methodus dandi relationes*, 1578), Giovanni Battista Codronchi (*Methodus testificandi*, 1597), and Fortunaus Fidelis (*De relationibus médicorum*, 1598).[14] Juan Fragoso's treatise was not the earliest publication on the subject but was the first for Spain. His work fits into the middle of this trend temporally and attempted, as others did, to succinctly discuss the variety of issues surgeons may be called upon for their expertise. Just as Díaz was not necessarily the first to write on many aspects of urology, so Fragoso was not the first to write on many of the topics he includes. Luis Lobera de Ávila, for example, discusses issues of fertility that would require some expertise to determine, including rare events such as superfetation and hermaphrodism, in his 1551 treatise, *Libro del regimiento de la salud y de la estirilidad de los hombres y mujeres y de las enfermedades de los niños y otras cosas utilísimas*. Dionisio Daza Chacón reflects on the importance of surgeons being able to give an accurate prognosis of wounds, not only for knowing how to proceed with treatment but also for providing legal testimony if asked, which seems to have been a common occurrence.[15] In fact, Fragoso mixes stories of his own experience with many accounts from other writers, authors including Ambroise Paré, Paracelsus, Girolamo Cardano, Giovanni da Vigo, Andres de Laguna, and Francisco Valles. Yet he also includes topics not discussed by others including poisonings, death from apoplexy, the examination of the health of enslaved people before their purchase, and a variety of sexual questions such as the determination of sodomy and the question of whether a woman can impregnate another woman.[16] The treatise is a mix of the mundane and the rare, issues that many surgeons may be asked to weigh in on and other things none are likely to ever encounter.

Fragoso's treatise first appeared in print around the same time that Francisco Díaz was called upon to give expert testimony in a very unusual legal case, that of Eleno/a de Céspedes.[17] This occurred in 1586 when Díaz was well established at court and on the cusp of publishing his work on urology, which received permission for publication in 1587 and appeared in 1588. In this particular case, Díaz's expertise in anatomy, particularly urogenital anatomy, was needed. Eleno de Céspedes applied for a marriage license in order to marry María del Caño. Céspedes, who had been raised female, but had shifted back and forth between identifying (dressing) as male or female, was by this time living as a man. The vicar, suspicious of his lack of facial hair or other "male" features, requested he be examined by doctors, which he readily agreed to. He successfully withstood examination from a number of doctors and surgeons, Francisco Díaz among them. Díaz, like all other doctors and surgeons involved in the case, examined Céspedes both visually and manually and then testified that he found no genital evidence that Céspedes could be a woman. The marriage was allowed to proceed, but this did not stop news or rumors from continuing to surround Céspedes, who was arrested along with María nearly a year later. The case wound up in Inquisition courts, where Céspedes was now accused of sorcery (used to convince everyone of his manhood) and insult to the sacrament of marriage. At this point, Céspedes, who was a licensed surgeon, began to make the case that s/he was a hermaphrodite. Céspedes claimed to have both male and female genitalia, with a penis that had been retained internally until adulthood, beginning to emerge with the strain of childbirth several years earlier. Though hermaphrodism was not discussed by Fragoso in his treatise on legal medicine, it was discussed by other medical writers, including Lobera de Ávila mentioned earlier, and Ambroise Paré. Thus, it was not an unheard of condition, even if extremely rare. It is notable that Céspedes owned a handful of medical books by this time, including Paré, and may have been using knowledge from them in this defense. In addition, Céspedes admitted to having "prepared certain remedies with wine and alcohol, and many other remedies and potions to see if I could close my woman's part."[18] Díaz and others rescinded their earlier testimonies, turning to sorcery for an explanation of how they had been fooled, and Céspedes was eventually convicted of both charges. Leaving aside the very complex issues of both sex and gender in this case, it remains a remarkable example of surgical expertise, albeit used for different purposes, on the part of both Díaz and Céspedes.

Fragoso asserts that he offered his treatise, as so many sixteenth-century surgeons similarly claim, at the demand of many surgeons who urged him to compile his knowledge for the greater good. Here we more clearly see Fragoso as an innovator, compiling knowledge from colleagues and his own experiences to expand the range of surgical expertise. In addition, Fragoso was the only Spanish surgeon and the earliest practicing surgeon in Europe to write treatises specifically on materia medica (of which he wrote three).[19] All others who wrote herbals, botanical studies, or materia medica studies were physicians, whether actively practicing or not. In Spain that includes such figures as Andrés Laguna, Francisco Hernández, Nicolas Monardes, and Simón de Tovar. The Englishman John Gerarde (d. 1612) was the only other practicing surgeon who wrote on plants. In offering his knowledge on legal questions, Fragoso likewise shows himself unique in his interests. He sought to professionalize the public image of surgeons as reliable medical-legal experts who could and would use their specialized knowledge of the body (and particularly of wounds) for the larger good of the community, providing the first Spanish treatise to specifically discuss various areas in which the expertise of the surgeon could be called upon in a court of law.

Gunpowder Wounds

Over the course of the sixteenth century, warfare became ubiquitous in parts of Europe, thanks in no small part to the great rivalry of Charles V and Francis I. Though gunpowder weapons had been developed sometime in the fourteenth century, such weapons came to dominate the battlefield in the sixteenth. Military surgeons then had to cope with new types of wounds, distinct from the cutting or penetrating wounds caused by arrows, swords, or other earlier weapons.[20] The debate that emerged over gunpowder wounds was one of theory as well as practice, tangled around the question of what gunpowder itself did to the body. By the turn of the sixteenth century, an increasing number of surgeons believed that gunpowder was poisonous, and wounds caused by gunshot needed to have that poison neutralized by cautery in order to prevent its spread throughout the body. Numerous surgeons added their voices to the debate on how to classify and treat this new problem, including Dionisio Daza Chacón.

Among early proponents of the belief in gunpowder poison were Hieronymus Brunschwig in a 1497 treatise and, much more influentially, Giovanni da Vigo, remembered both for his role as surgeon to Pope Julius II and for his influential text, *Practica in arte chirurgica copiosa* (1514). This was followed by a second, more condensed text, *Practica compendiosa* (1517) a few years later. In discussing gunshot wounds, he described the poison of gunpowder as dangerous not just to the wound site but also potentially spreading throughout the body, causing much more significant problems. In advocating that the best means of stopping this spread was cauterizing the wound, through either actual (burning iron) or "potential" (boiling oil) means, Vigo was returning to a practice more common in the ancient world and advocated by many Islamic surgical texts. An ancient treatment for a new form of wound. Cautery as a form of treatment for wounds, however, had largely disappeared in medieval Europe, so Vigo's advocating for it was in fact a turn toward older authorities to reintroduce a little-used method of treatment.[21] Vigo's authoritative text became enormously popular, undergoing more than forty editions, with translation into French, English, Spanish, and German.[22]

Many other surgeons of the early sixteenth century quickly rejected the theory of gunpowder poisoning wounds, including Berengario da Carpi (1518), Paracelsus (1536), and, most famously, Ambroise Paré whose 1545 text, *La methode de traycter leys playes faictes par hacquebutes et altres bastons à feu*, detailed his experiences on the battlefield and his experiments in treating gunshot wounds. Paré, who remains the best-known surgeon of the era, carefully framed his argument for discarding the traditional use of boiling oil for gunshot wounds as one of necessity—overwhelming numbers of wounded meant that the oil ran out and he was forced to try something else:

> At last I wanted oyl, and was constrained in steed thereof, to apply a digestive of yolkes of egges, oyle of Roses, and Turpentine. In the night I could not sleepe in quiet, fearing some default in not cauterizing, that I should finde those to whom I had not used the burning oyle dead impoysoned; which made me rise very early to visit them, where beyond my expectation I found those to whom I had applyed my digestive medicine, to feele little paine, and their wounds without inflammation or tumor, having rested reasonable well in the night: the others to whom was used the sayd burning oyle, I found them feverish, with great paine and tumor about the edges of their wounds. And then I resolved with my selfe never so cruelly, to burn poore men wounded with gunshot.[23]

Paré has received much attention over the centuries for being the first to publish his experiences and for describing them so carefully. His willingness to reject traditional treatment in the face of experimental evidence has made him the face of "modern" experimental surgery. Thus, as he describes it, he performed an unplanned (and even reluctant) experiment but then made use of his observation of results that provided a new way of healing more successfully. Paré, however, was neither the first nor the only military surgeon of his era to question Vigo and turn to other methods, as demonstrated by Paré himself. His text immediately goes on to recount his lengthy efforts over the next two years to obtain from an (unnamed) fellow surgeon ("who had fame above all others") at Turin his secret recipe for a special oil used to treat such gunshot wounds.[24] This is the famous "oil of puppies," which Paré subsequently shared in his text despite also recounting his promises to guard it as secret. Indeed, many surgeons were likewise wary of or rejected cautery for wounds, while others experimented with their own formulations of healing oils. These included the Italians Bartolomeo Maggi (1477–c. 1552), Leonardo Botallo (c.1519–87), and Leonardo Fioravanti (1517–88), and Englishmen Thomas Gale (1507–86) and William Clowes (1543–1604). But the lines of accepting or rejecting cautery were not always so clear cut. Giovanni Francesco Rota (1520–58) and Ippolito Boschi (c.1540–1612), for example, though rejecting the use of cautery for gunshot nonetheless retained the view that gunpowder was indeed poisonous, while Hans von Gersdorff advocated cautery despite rejecting the proposition that gunpowder acted as a poison.[25] The debates over how gunpowder affected the body and how to treat these wounds continued through the century. The treatises of Alfonso Ferri (1552, who embraced the poison theory), Rota, and Botallo (1555 and 1560, both of whom rejected it) were reprinted together as late as 1583.[26]

The most prominent Spanish voice in this debate was Dionisio Daza Chacón, a military surgeon who offered his own experiences and theory in his 1580 text. Daza Chacón acknowledges and reflects at length on the debates of the previous half century, adding his own accumulated experiences from the past four decades of practice. He is disdainful of the weapons themselves, calling the arquebus a "wretched and pernicious weapon, destroyer of life and honor, and exalter of weak men."[27] Daza Chacón makes clear his knowledge of the debates on the nature of these wounds, citing many of the earlier referenced earlier works: Vigo, Ferri, Paré, Botallo. He rejects the idea of gunpowder being poisonous because it

> is made from three things, one part sulfur, one part charcoal and ten parts saltpeter…not only are none of these poisonous, they have no association of poison because not only are they used externally for many diseases, but are taken internally as well, to great effect.[28]

He goes on to reject any "occult" or hidden process by which such innocuous (even helpful) ingredients could become venomous when mixed.

Of the chapters he devotes to gunpowder wounds, the longest is that on the treatment of them. The chapters come at the end of the third (and last) book, in which he addresses wounds in particular parts of the body. He uses a traditional organization in this section, beginning with the head (separately addressing the skull, eyes, nose, ears, and so forth) and moving downwards through the body. After chapters addressing wounds to all the different internal organs of the abdomen, he turns to wounds made by the arquebus. The final four chapters of the book address the history of the arquebus, whether such wounds are poisoned, the symptoms of gunpowder wounds, and finally the treatment of them. In the midst of this chapter, he recounts his early experience on the battlefield under Charles V in the 1540s. At the 1544 siege of Saint Dizier, an Italian surgeon who he calls "Micer Bartolomeo" arrived at camp and began treating the wounded quite differently than the Spaniards. This Italian surgeon, who Daza Chacón describes as "very learned and experienced" has been identified as likely Bartolomeo Maggi (1477?–1552), who along with lecturing in surgery at the University of Bologna later became the personal physician to Pope Julius III.[29] Maggi had also rejected the notion of gunshot as poisonous, though his treatise would only be published posthumously in 1552. For Daza Chacón, the results were immediately clear. This alternate method allowed patients to heal more quickly and with less pain, so Daza Chacón quickly embraced it.[30] Notably, this was in the same war (though on the opposite side) as Paré recounts in his text. The difference, of course, was that Paré published his text soon thereafter, while Daza Chacón waited until retirement, writing his nearly decades later. It is telling, though, that even seventy years after Vigo's text and forty after Paré's, Daza Chacón still felt it worthwhile to recount his own battlefield experiences and weigh in on the debate. The treating of gunshot wounds "softly" with unguents rather than cautery was framed by Paré, Daza Chacón, and other surgeons as born of necessity and proved by experience.

New Diseases

The sixteenth-century battlefield offered a welter of new problems for surgeons, learned or not. Increased warfare and the use of mercenary troops meant more bodies gathered together from different regions and generally housed in unsanitary conditions. This combination of crowded conditions and the movement of large groups of soldiers as they gathered, fought, and later disbanded resulted in outbreaks of disease. It is no surprise that the two new diseases of the late fifteenth century, typhus and the Great Pox (morbo gálico, mal frances, or las bubas in Spanish), both first gained recognition among soldiers at war. Whether these diseases were truly new to Europeans, and the intertwined question of retrospective diagnosis (for example, whether what they diagnosed as morbo gálico was the same disease we diagnose as syphilis) are complex issues that have absorbed many scholars.[31] For our purposes, it matters only that many patients experiencing these diseases and medical men treating them believed them to be new, which engendered many of the debates over causation and treatment that surgeons participated in. How to refer to diseases in the past remains a fraught question for modern scholars. In an effort to remain both historically accurate and sensitive to these debates, I am using the modern English term typhus as it is largely accepted by scholars as an umbrella term to bring together what Spaniards had many names for tabardillo, tabardete, fiebre punticular, fiebre lenticular, las pintas, and others. On the other hand, I use the Spanish morbo gálico, as this was a standard term used by nearly all Spanish Renaissance practitioners, while the modern term syphilis remains contested as an equivalent.[32]

In turning to examine surgeons and disease, the hybridity of the médico y cirujano becomes clear, as learned surgeons worked alongside physicians in not only diagnosing and treating these diseases but also participating in debates about them and publishing treatises on them. It is not at all surprising that surgeons treated plague, typhus, and morbo gálico, for they all manifested visibly on the skin in buboes, rashes, and sores. Surgeons had long been called upon to lance abscesses and apply ointments to all manner of skin ailments. Yet sixteenth-century surgeons went beyond simple discussions of treatment, participating in debates about the nature of these diseases: what conditions gave rise to them, whether they were contagious or not, whether the ancients had in fact treated and discussed these same conditions (or at least something similar). In this way, they positioned themselves as knowledgeable experts not just in their manual skills of treatment but also in their deeper understanding of medical theory and the body within its environment.

Learned surgeons included discussions of disease within their surgical texts in various ways. Those, like Bartolomé Hidalgo de Agüero, Juan Fragoso, and Juan Calvo who included antidotaries in their texts included various specific treatments (internal and external) for all these diseases, as well as topical applications for the usual range of sores or rashes. Others included discussions of disease either as separate chapters, books, or treatises within their texts, such as Andrés Alcázar's final two books on morbo gálico (twenty-eight chapters) and plague (twenty-one chapters), Francisco Arceo's four chapters on morbo gálico in Book II, Bartolomé Hidalgo de Agüero's chapter on morbo gálico and two appended treatises on plague and typhus, and Juan Calvo's added treatise on morbo gálico. Other surgeons published treatises separate from their surgical texts, such as Antonio Pérez's 1568 treatise on plague and Andrés de León's 1605 treatise on morbo gálico. Regardless of the structure of their writings, surgeons worked to add their voices alongside physicians to advise on disease.

Typhus and Plague

Typhus became familiar to Europeans in the sixteenth century. The disease itself is quite ancient and has been pointed to as a possible culprit for the plague of Athens famously described by Thucydides.[33] Other historians have found scattered references to what may have been typhus from the eleventh century onward. For example, Juan de Avignon (Moses ben Samuel), a fourteenth-century Jewish convert who practiced medicine in Seville for a time, refers to outbreaks of tabardillo in that city in his text, *Sevillana Medicina*.[34] This work was not known until the mid-sixteenth century, however, when it was published by Nicolas Monardes. Outbreaks among Spanish soldiers in 1489 during the Wars of Granada (1482–92) and in Italy in the early decades of the sixteenth century are most often acknowledged as the beginning of verifiable outbreaks.[35] The earliest detailed description of typhus as a distinct disease is credited to Italian physician Girolamo Fracastoro in his 1546 text *De contagione et contagiosis morbis et eorum curatione*.[36] Thus, typhus was (and essentially still is) seen as a new disease in the sixteenth century, one born of warfare and poverty.

Typhus and plague were intertwined in the sixteenth century, seen often as two sides of the same coin of pestilence. Both contagions arose in waves, believed to originate from and spread through various means: poverty and bad diet, miasmas (corruption of the air), and infected clothing or bedding. The differences between them, however, were important. Typhus was viewed as pernicious but not dire; plague remained far more feared. For typhus, a more "common" pestilence, there was no need to erect the elaborate public health measures that plague required. Those public health measures, including closing city gates, limiting travel, and setting up isolation hospitals, had real and often devastating economic effects for residents. Thus, untangling the two and distinguishing between them became of utmost importance. In the late sixteenth century, surgeons were central to efforts to better understand and clearly diagnose typhus. They worked and published alongside physicians, asserting their experience-based expertise in two main formats. During outbreaks of disease, civic leaders in many cities gathered local physicians and surgeons to give expert opinions on the level of pestilential threat. Surgeons and physicians (and sometimes apothecaries) reported on what cases they had seen, what form of pestilence seemed to be circulating, and what public health measures should be enacted. In the aftermath of outbreaks, both physicians and surgeons published treatises on plague and typhus, offering their views on and experiences with each disease.

In April 1582, for example, as Seville faced a growing epidemic, the city council called together leading physicians, surgeons (some identified as médico y cirujano and others merely as cirujano), and apothecaries to ascertain the nature of the epidemic. Among the fourteen physicians and surgeons who testified to the city council was Bartolomé Hidalgo de Agüero, along with other well-known figures, including physician Nicolas Monardes, physician and surgeon Francisco Sánchez de Oropesa, physician Alonso Valdés, and physician Alonso Díez Daza. There was, however, no clear agreement among them. Some saw signs of plague in their patients, others only ordinary fevers and swellings. Several argued that while some patients did exhibit signs of a "venomous" contagion, the dangers of officially acknowledging a plague epidemic and enacting anti-contagion measures seemed to them to outweigh the dangers of disease spread. Several weeks later, the epidemic unabated, the city council again called in medical practitioners, some who had testified earlier and others who had not. Once again, while the mix of physicians and surgeons all agreed there was a contagion running through the city, their predictions of how dangerous it was (whether it was true plague or a milder pestilence) and their views of how the city leaders should respond were varied. [37] Such discussions among medical men and city leaders, sometimes simple testimonials and sometimes heated debates, occurred in cities throughout Spain as local authorities sought to control public health in their jurisdictions.[38] In these discussions, learned surgeons participated on equal footing with physicians, not only as eyewitnesses to what patients were suffering but also as experts in the interpretation of symptoms and theoretical distinctions between diseases.

Surgeons also wrote about diseases with equal experience and knowledge as physicians. As surgeons asserted increasing expertise and knowledge of diseases, physicians did not yield that expertise to them. In surveying these treatises on disease, it becomes increasingly difficult to distinguish between physicians and surgeons. The earliest Spanish text on typhus was not from Spain but instead was published in Mexico City. Francisco Bravo's 1570 text, *Opera Medicinalia*, contained four distinct treatises, one of which focused on *tabardete*. Just a few years later, texts began to appear in Spain, including three published in 1574. Physicians Luis de Toro, Alfonso López de Corella, and Luis Mercado each produced Latin treatises on the disease. Luis Mercado (1525–1611) was at the time an eminent professor of medicine at the University of Valladolid, though within a few years he rose to become royal physician to Philip II and Protomédico. His interest in writing about this disease (as well as plague and morbo gálico, which he also later wrote treatises on) reflects the deep interest that these diseases still held for physicians as well as learned surgeons. Over the next three decades, treatises continued to proliferate from both physicians and learned surgeons. Nicolas Bocangelino included typhus (*fiebre punticular*) in his vernacular treatise *Libro de las enfermedades malignas y pestilentes, causas, pronosticos, curacion, y preservacion*, and Bartolomé Hidalgo de Agüero appended two separate treatises to the end of his surgical compendium, one on plague and the other on typhus.

At the end of the century, in response to a severe and widespread epidemic, often now known as the Atlantic Plague (1596–1602), surgeons once again participated in debates with physicians, writing new treatises in the aftermath.[39] In 1599, the royal physician Cristóbal Pérez de Herrera published a work on plague raising questions about treatment—the use of purgatives and the type of diet prescribed in particular. In response, the Council of Castile convened a meeting of four royal court physicians (led by Alfonso Zamudio de Alfaro, who was then royal physician and Protomédico), three court surgeons (including the learned surgeon Antonio Pérez), and three other prominent physicians. From this meeting came little agreement among the men, but several publications on plague, including Pérez's. A second group, which met in Seville this same year, likewise included prominent local figures, both physicians and surgeons.[40] This meeting produced no less than seven separate treatises from its constituent members.

Morbo Gálico or the Great Pox

The disease that erupted at the siege of Naples in 1493 came to be known by many different names: *lues venerea*, *morbus gallicus*, the Great Pox, the French disease, the Neapolitan disease, morbo gálico, and so forth. Andrés de León, in his 1605 treatise on morbo gálico, includes a list of names Spaniards used:

> some [call it] the French disease, others Spanish scabies, others Neapolitan disease, others measles from the Indies: the Portuguese [call it] Castilian disease, the native Americans of Portugal [call it] the Portuguese disease...others [call it] the serpentine disease of Española and in Spain they call it bubas.[41]

Following Girolamo Fracastoro's 1530 publication, it also became known as syphilis. This welter of names gave rise to important questions that remained debated for centuries (and in some cases are still debated by historians today). Did these names all refer to the same disease? Was this something new or merely an older disease(s) now called by new names? If new, why or how did it arise?

The questions of origin and identity were closely tied to those of treatment and remained at the forefront of medical writing for centuries. The earliest writings on the Pox in Europe were from physicians who asserted intellectual authority, participating in disputations and publishing learned treatises.[42] The rapid and continued spread of the disease, however, meant that while medical men continued to debate and publish, sufferers turned to practitioners of all levels of education and training in hopes of relief. Like plague and typhus, morbo gálico remained contested ground among physicians, surgeons, and empirics over its origins, means of spread, and best treatment regimes.[43]

Spanish surgeons who wrote about morbo gálico were doing so nearly a century after its initial eruption, and their work reflects the unsettled nature of these questions. That surgeons tackled not only the treatment of morbo gálico but also the questions of its origins and nature (how it spread) reflects their erudition: they showed familiarity with ancient works that could be used to attest to either the antiquity or novelty of this disease, an equal or greater familiarity with the arguments of a wide range of recent or contemporary authors, and firsthand experience in the efficacy of various remedies for the disease.

The longest discussions of morbo gálico were from Andrés Alcázar (Book 5 of his surgical treatise, composed of twenty-eight chapters) Francisco Arceo (four chapters in Book II of his surgical treatise), Juan Calvo (a treatise of twenty-five chapters appended to his surgical text), Andrés de León (a stand-alone treatise of fifty-nine chapters), and Juan Fragoso (a discussion of several pages in the Antidotario of his surgical text, under the heading "Polvos contra el mal Frances"). All except Arceo begin their treatises with a discussion of the disease's origins, recounting arguments that had long been made by others both for its antiquity and its modernity.[44] Like their colleagues across Europe, those who argued it was not new pointed to another confusing variety of conditions discussed in ancient and Islamic treatises, including *lichines*, *mentagra*, *asafati*, which might encompass the disease then being experienced.[45] The four who discuss origins all spend a surprising amount of time detailing two different theories of the disease's more recent origins, though only Calvo actually believed this to be a new disease. The two theories recounted were that it originated from the New World, brought to Europe by the men on Columbus's early voyage, or that it had arisen as a result of cannibalism that had occurred among soldiers at the siege of Naples. [46] While this cannibalism was considered to be an inadvertent act—the soldiers who began to suffer the disease were unaware that desperate and unscrupulous sutlers had scavenged human flesh along with animal flesh to use in their dishes—the deep immorality of it created corruption within their bodies, flowering into a disease that could then be passed to others in a variety of ways. Juan Calvo is the only one who gives these theories of a modern emergence credibility, though he merges the two theories in a unique way. He doesn't deny the terrible immorality of cannibalism, nor that it had occurred at Naples, but argues that this particular instance of it had not resulted in a new disease. In fact, he asserts that in many wars, "soldiers have, without knowing it, eaten such awful things, the meat of horses as well as humans" without such a disease arising.[47] Thus, he turns to history and the fact that in no previous wars where conditions were dire did anyone suffer a similar outbreak of corruptive disease. Instead, Calvo argued that the disease had arrived in Europe from the Americas, where it had arisen as a result of cannibalistic practices that were commonly enacted there by choice.[48] Inadvertent cannibalism (or that born of dreadful necessity) was not sufficient grounds to cause such corruption, but deliberate and purposeful cannibalism could. Early chroniclers of the Indies had portrayed societies steeped in immorality, including pervasive cannibalism, which Calvo then linked to the timing of when this new disease erupted, bringing the two theories together.

The discussions of morbo gálico are rife with the theoretical and practical. These learned surgeons embrace the idea that this disease was no mere humoral imbalance, but a corruption in all parts of the body, down into the very bones themselves.[49] They refer not only to the work of respected physicians Luis Mercado and Francisco Valles but also to that of Nicolò Leoniceno, Girolamo Fallopio, Nicolò Massa, and Giovanni da Vigo. They suggest varying treatments, depending on the pervasiveness of corruption. Fragoso and Alcázar both divide the disease into different "kinds" or stages, offering various treatments for each. As Fragoso states, "[T]he remedies for this illness are diverse, according to the species and variety of symptoms, each of which requires a particular approach."[50] The surgeon must know how to read the signs of the body to determine which kind of corruption the patient suffered and therefore how best to treat them. Calvo disagreed with the idea of different types of infection, specifically referring to "Fernelio [Jean Fernel], Alcaçar y Fragoso" as among those who incorrectly do so.[51] Calvo insisted that as this was a single disease, such distinctions were unnecessary. In offering a range of treatments, each surgeon provides his own theoretical framework for when and why these were useful treatments. Fragoso's discussion of the disease is part of his Antidotary, where he offers more discussion about the disease than treatment, but he does include a range of compound recipes. Calvo, offering recipes for different syrups (jarabes), divides the section into "those of a phlegmatic termperament," "for melancholics," and "for cholerics."[52] In addressing treatment, learned surgeons discuss the preparation and use of the range of treatments then common in Europe: china root, guaiacum (palo santo), sarsaparilla (çarçaparilla), and mercury treatments. Some, such as Bartolomé Hidalgo de Agüero, reflect on the waning popularity of milder treatments of guaiacum and sarsaparilla, arguing for the "stronger" cures necessary to root out such a deep-seated corruption.[53]

That learned surgeons incorporated discussions of an increasingly broad range of topics reflects both their deeper intellectual training and their reconceptualizing of medical practice to further shift or entirely remove the boundaries between types of healers. Familiarity with ancient and medieval medical theories enabled them to expand the expertise of surgeons, applying the art of medicine to many new issues.

Notes

1 Juan Calvo, *Primera y segunda parte de la cirugia uniuersal y particular del cuerpo humano* (Madrid: Diego Flamenco, 1626), 2.

2 See for example, Francisco Díaz, *Compendio de chirurgia: En el qual de trata de todas las cosas tocantes la theorica y pratica della* (Madrid, 1575), fols. 2–3; Calvo, *Cirugia uniuersal*, 1626, 1–3; Juan Fragoso, *Cirugia universal ... y mas otros tres tratados ... El primero es, una summa de proposiciones contraciertos avisos de cirugia. El segundo, de las declaraciones acerca de diversas heridas y muertos. El tercero, de los Aphorismos de Hyppocrates tocantes a cirugia*, 1592, fols. 1–2.

3 Michael R. McVaugh, *The Rational Surgery of the Middle Ages*, Micrologus' Library 15 (Firenze: SISMEL-Edizione del Galluzzo, 2006), 135–74.

4 See, for example, Juan Fragoso, *Cirugia uniuersal, aora nueuamenta añadida* (1627), 14–19, 437–39, 545; Juan Calvo, *Primera y segunda parte de la cirugia uniuersal y particular del cuerpo humano* (Madrid, 1674), 469–74, 244–51, Hidalgo de Agüero, *Thesoro de la verdadera cirugía y vía particular contra la común*, 207v–09v, 118.

5 "Por que aunque Laguna Medico Espanol doctissimo, y el Dotor Romano escrivieron de carnosidades…fue tan sucintamente que apenas por ello se puede entender que cosa sea el mal. Y si Galeno y otros autores graves escrivieron de las enfermedades de rinones, y vexiga fue en differentes tratados, salpicando y no reduciendolo a una obra sola." Francisco Díaz, *Tratado, nuevamente impresso, de todas las enfermedades de los riñones, vexiga, y carnosidades de la verga y urina: dividido en tres libros* (Madrid, 1588), n.p.

6 William Eamon, *Science and the Secrets of Nature: Books of Secrets in Medieval and Early Modern Culture* (Princeton, N.J: Princeton University Press, 1994); Elaine Leong and Alisha Rankin, eds., *Secrets and Knowledge in Medicine and Science, 1500–1800* (New York: Routledge, 2011).

7 "[N]o han de faltar murmuradores…Pero suplicote Letor pijssimo, si alguna cosa no te pareciere dina de salir a luz, se reconpense con muchas nuevas utilissimas" Díaz, *Tratado*, Prologo al lector.

8 Díaz, 320–2; Michele L Clouse, *Medicine, Government and Public Health in Philip II's Spain: Shared Interests, Competing Authorities* (Burlington, VT: Ashgate, 2011), 91–8.

9 Francisco Sánchez de Oropesa, *Discurso del doctor Francisco Sánchez de Oropesa para averiguar q[ue] mal de urina sea el q[ue] padece Diego Anriquez Leon su amigo i conpadre: en que incidentemente se tratan las cosas que parecieron dificultosas i de mas consideraciõ cerca de la essencia, causas, señales i cura de todos los males deste genero…* (en casa de Iuan de Leon, 1594).

10 "En el año de 1588, aqui in Madrid, aviendo palabras un hombre con una muger, hallaron, que el hombre murio repentinamente, y la justicia hizo junta de Cirujanos, para saber de que avia muerto" Juan Fragoso, *Cirugia universal, aora nuevamente emendada, y añadida* (Madrid: Viuda de Alonso Gómez, 1586), 298.

11 "Tratado secundo de las declaraciones que han de hazer los Cirujanos acerca de diversas enfermedades y muchas maneras de muertes que suceden" Fragoso, *Cirugia universal*, fol. 286v.

12 Peter Volk and Hans Jurgen Warlo, "The Role of Medical Experts in Court Proceedings in the Medieval Town," in *International Symposium on Society, Medicine and the Law, Jerusalem, March 1972* (New York: Elsevier Scientific Publishing Co, 1973), 101–16; Alessandro Simili, "The Beginnings of Forensic Medicine in Bologna," in *International Symposium on Society, Medicine and the Law, Jerusalem, March 1972* (New York: Elsevier Scientific

Publishing Co, 1973), 91–100; Katharine Park, "The Criminal and the Saintly Body: Autopsy and Dissection in Renaissance Italy," *Renaissance Quarterly* 47, no. 1 (1994): 1–33, https://doi.org/10.2307/2863109; Mercedes Gallent Marco, "Precedentes medievales de la medicina legal: la 'dessospitació' en el Reino de Valencia," *Saitabi: Revista de La Facultat de Geografia i Història* 50 (2000): 11–28.

13 Gallent Marco, "Precedentes medievales de la medicina legal"; Michael R. McVaugh, *Medicine before the Plague: Practitioners and Their Patients in the Crown of Aragon, 1285–1345* (Cambridge: Cambridge University Press, 2002), 207–18.

14 Erwin H. Ackerknecht, "Early History of Legal Medicine," in *Legacies in Law and Medicine*, ed. Chester R. Burns (New York: Science History Publications, 1977), 249–71; Silvia De Renzi, "Medical Expertise, Bodies, and the Law in Early Modern Courts," *Isis* 98, no. 2 (2007): 315–22, https://doi.org/10.1086/518191; Catherine Crawford, "Legalizing Medicine: Early Modern Legal Systems and the Growth of Medico-Legal Knowledge," in *Legal Medicine in History*, ed. Michael Clark and Catherine Crawford (New York: Cambridge University Press, 1994).

15 Jacinto Corbella, "El crecimiento del saber medico legal en España en el siglo XVI," *Asclepio: Revista de Historia de La Medicina y de La Ciencia* 30–31 (1978-79): 328, 334.

16 Antonio Carreras Panchón, *La obra de Juan de Villarreal y otros estudios historico-medicos*, Cuadernos de Historia de La Medicina Española. Monografias 33 (Salamanca: Ediciones Universidad de Salamanca, 1978), 33.

17 The Inquisition case which brought charges against Cespedes is detailed in Richard L. Kagan and Abigail Dyer, eds., *Inquisitorial Inquiries: Brief Lives of Secret Jews and Other Heretics* (Baltimore, MD: Johns Hopkins University Press, 2011), 64–87 though not Díaz's specific testimony. Díaz's involvement in the case is discussed in Emilio Maganto Pavón, "La Intervención Del Dr. Francisco Díaz En El Proceso Inquisitorial Contra Elena/o de Céspedes, Una Cirujana Transexual Condenada Por La Inquisición de Toledo En 1587," *Archivos Españoles de Urología* 60, no. 8 (2007): 873–86.

18 Kagan and Dyer, *Inquisitorial Inquiries*, 72.

19 Juan Fragoso, *Catalogus simplicium medicamentorum* (Alcalá de Henares: P. Robles & J. Villanoua, 1566); Juan Fragoso, *Discurso de las cosas aromaticas, arboles y frutales y de otras muchas medicinas simples que se traen de la India Oriental y que siruen al vso de medicina* (Madrid: en casa de Francisco Sanchez, 1572); Juan Fragoso, *De succedaneis medicamentis liber denuo auctus…Ejusdem animadversiones, in quamplurima medicamenta composita, quoru[m] est usus in hispanicis officinis* (Madrid, 1575).

20 Kelly R DeVries, "Military Surgical Practice and the Advent of Gunpowder Weaponry," *Canadian Bulletin of Medical History* 7, no. 2 (1990): 134–6, https://doi.org/10.3138/cbmh.7.2.131; J. R. Hale, *War and Society in Renaissance Europe, 1450–1620* (New York: St. Martin's Press, 1985), 46–52.

21 DeVries, "Military Surgical Practice and the Advent of Gunpowder Weaponry."

22 Arturo Castiglioni, *A History of Medicine*, trans. E. B. Krumbhaar, 2nd ed. (New York: Knopf, 1947), 470.

23 Ambroise Paré, *The Apologie and Treatise of Ambroise Paré: Containing the Voyages Made into Divers Places, with Many of His Writings upon Surgery*, Classics of Science (Chicago: University of Chicago Press, 1952), 23–4.

24 Paré, 24.

25 J.S. Taylor, "United States Naval Medical Bulletin. v. 15, 1921," *United States Naval Medical Bulletin. v. 15, 1921* XV, no. 3 (1921): 575–80; Charles Singer, "The Early Treatment of Gunshot Wounds," *The Quarterly Review* 226, no. 449 (1916): 464–9; William Eamon, "The Legend of Ambroise Paré and the 'Liberation' of Surgery," *William Eamon* (blog), accessed July 11, 2020, https://williameamon.com/?p=297.

26 Alfonso Ferri, Giovanni Francesco Rota, and Leonardo Botallo, *De curandis vulneribus sclopetorum tractatus singulares* (Antverpiae: Ex officina Arnoldi Coninx, 1583).

27 Dionisio Daza Chacón, *Segunda parte de la pratica y teorica de cirugia en romance y en latin, que trata de todas las heridas en general, y en particular* (por la viuda de Alonso Martin, a costa de Domingo Gonçalez, 1626), 338.

28 "De tres cosas se haze la polvora, de una parte de acufre, y otra de carbon de salze, y deiz partes de salitre…ninguna de ellas, no solo no es venenosa, pero no tiene sospecha de veneno, porque no solo se aplican or deferua para muchas enferemedades, pero se toman, y administran por dentro para muchos afectos" Dionisio Daza Chacón, *Pratica y teorica de cirugia en romance y en latin* (por Francisco Cipres, 1673), 258.

29 Charles Donald O'Malley, *Andreas Vesalius of Brussels, 1514–1564* (Berkeley: University of California Press, 1965), 205.

30 Daza Chacón, *Segunda parte*, 344–5.

31 While modern scientific analysis of human remains, including skeletal and aDNA analysis, have greatly advanced our knowledge of the presence of disease in the past, retrospective diagnosis remains an often-tricky issue. See Andrew Cunningham, "Identifying Disease in the Past: Cutting the Gordian Knot," *Asclepio* 54, no. 1 (2002): 13–34, https://doi.org/10.3989/asclepio.2002.v54.i1.133; Jon Arrizabalaga, "Problematizing Retrospective Diagnosis in the History of Disease," *Asclepio: Revista de Historia de La Medicina y de La Ciencia* 54, no. 1 (2002): 51–70. The origins of syphilis, in particular, remains hotly debated among biomedical scientists. Some recent studies reflecting arguments for both the Old World (pre-Columbian) and New World origins of syphilis would include Ivana Anteric et al., "Which Theory for the Origin of Syphilis Is True?," *The Journal of Sexual Medicine* 11, no. 12 (2014): 3112–18, https://doi.org/10.1111/jsm.12674; George J. Armelagos, Molly K. Zuckerman, and Kristin N. Harper, "The Science Behind Pre-Columbian Evidence of Syphilis in Europe: Research by Documentary," *Evolutionary Anthropology: Issues, News, and Reviews* 21, no. 2 (2012): 50–7, https://doi.org/10.1002/evan.20340; Kristin N. Harper et al., "The Origin and Antiquity of Syphilis Revisited: An Appraisal of Old World Pre-Columbian Evidence for Treponemal Infection," *American Journal of Physical Anthropology* 146, no. S53 (2011): 99–133, https://doi.org/10.1002/ajpa.21613; Carme Rissech et al., "A Roman Skeleton with Possible Treponematosis in the North-East of the Iberian Peninsula: A Morphological and Radiological Study," *International Journal of Osteoarchaeology* 23, no. 6 (November 2013): 651–63, https://doi.org/10.1002/oa.1293; Don Walker et al., "Evidence of Skeletal Treponematosis from the Medieval Burial Ground of St. Mary Spital, London, and Implications for the Origins of the Disease in Europe: Skeletal Treponematosis from St. Mary Spital," *American Journal of Physical Anthropology* 156, no. 1 (2015): 90–101, https://doi.org/10.1002/ajpa.22630. There is far less literature, either historical or scientific on typhus, though it is one of several epidemic diseases cited by some as the cause of the 5th century BCE "plague of Athens." See Thomas E. Morgan, "Plague or Poetry? Thucydides on the Epidemic at Athens," *Transactions of the American Philological Association* 124 (1994): 197–209, https://doi.org/10.2307/284291.

32 Jon Arrizabalaga has written a great deal on this. See Arrizabalaga, "Problematizing Retrospective Diagnosis in the History of Disease"; Jon Arrizabalaga, "Medical Causes of Death in Preindustrial Europe: Some Historiographical Considerations," *Journal of the History of Medicine and Allied Sciences* 54 (1999): 241–60.

33 Jean-Noël Biraben, "Diseases in Europe: Equilibrium and Breakdown of the Pathocenosis," in *Western Medical Thought from Antiquity to the Middle Ages*, ed. Mirko D. Grmek and Bernardino Fantini, trans. Antony Shugaar (Cambridge, MA: Harvard University Press, 1998), 325; Robert J. Littman, "The Plague of Athens: Epidemiology and Paleopathology," *The Mount Sinai Journal of Medicine, New York* 76, no. 5 (October 2009): 456–67, https://doi.org/10.1002/msj.20137.

34 Juan de Aviñón, *Sevillana Medicina: que trata el modo conservativo y curativo de los que habitan en… Sevilla (1545)* (Sevilla: Enrique Rasco, 1885), 33–8. The work was written in 1418 and later published by Nicolas Monardes in 1545.

35 August Hirsch, *Handbook of Geographical and Historical Pathology*, vol. I (New Sydenham Society, 1883), 546–9; Joaquín de Villalba y Guitarte, *Epidemiología española o Historia cronológica de las pestes, contagios, epidemias y epizootias que han acaecido en España desde la venida de las cartagineses hasta el año 1801: con noticia de algunas otras enfermedades que han*

sufrido los españoles en otros reynos, y de los autores nacionales que han escrito sobre esta materia... (Madrid, 1802), 69, 110; Juan Ignacio Carmona García, *Enfermedad y sociedad en los primeros tiempos modernos* (Sevilla: Secretariado de Publicaciones de la Universidad de Sevilla, 2005), 77–80; Hans Zinsser, *Rats, Lice, & History: Being a Study in Biography, Which, after Twelve Preliminary Chapters Indispensable for the Preparation of the Lay Reader, Deals with the Life History of Typhus Fever...* (Boston: Little, Brown and Company, 1963), 240–64.

36 Carmona García, *Enfermedad y sociedad en los primeros tiempos modernos*, 79.

37 The testimonials are in the Archivo Municipal de Sevilla, Seccion 13, siglo XVI, tomo 6, ff. 83–93 and 272–6. See also the discussions in Kristy Wilson Bowers, *Plague and Public Health in Early Modern Seville*, Rochester Studies in Medical History (Rochester, NY: University of Rochester Press, 2013), 37–8, 42–3; Alexandra Parma Cook and Noble David Cook, *The Plague Files: Crisis Management in Sixteenth-Century Seville* (Baton Rouge: Louisiana State University Press, 2009), 238–45, 252–5; Carmona García, *Enfermedad y sociedad en los primeros tiempos modernos*, 81–5.

38 Ruth MacKay, *Life in a Time of Pestilence* (New York: Cambridge University Press, 2019), 225–6; María del Carmen Gonzalez Muñoz, "Epidemias y enfermedades en Talavera de La Reina (SS. XVI y XVII)," *Hispania* 126 (1974): 154–5; Antonio Carreras Panchón, "Dos testimonios sobre la epidemia de peste de 1599 En Valladolid," *Asclepio: Revista de Historia de La Medicina y de La Ciencia* 25 (1973): 356.

39 Bernard Vincent, "La peste atlántica de 1596–1602," *Asclepio; Archivo Iberoamericano De Historia De La Medicina Y Antropologia Medica* 28 (1976): 5–25; Alfonso Arráez Tolosa, "El paso de la epidemia de la peste atlántica de 1596–1602 por Almansa," *Al-Basit* 63 (2018): 175–214; MacKay, *Life in a Time of Pestilence.*

40 Antonio Hernández Morejón, *Historia Bibliográfica de la Medicina Española (1842–1852)* IV, 69–73, http://147.156.5.138/Morejon_Chinchilla/; Villalba y Guitarte, *Epidemiología española o Historia cronológica de las pestes, contagios, epidemias y epizootias que han acaecido en España desde la venida de las cartagineses hasta el año 1801*, 231–3.

41 "[U]nos mal Frances, otros sarna Española, otros mal Napolitano, otros sarampion de las Indias: los Portugueses mal de Castilla, los Indios de Portugal, mal Portugues...otros morbo serpentino de la Isla Española, y en España bubas." Andrés de León, *Practico de morbo gallico, en el quel se contiene el origen y conocimiento della enfermedad, y el mejor modo de curarla* (Valladolid, 1605), 3.

42 Jon Arrizabalaga, John Henderson, and R. K French, *The Great Pox: The French Disease in Renaissance Europe* (New Haven, CT: Yale University Press, 1997); Roger French and Jon Arrizabalaga, "Coping with the French Disease: University Practitioners' Strategies and Tactics in the Transition from the Fifteenth to the Sixteenth Century," in *Medicine from the Black Death to the French Disease*, ed. Roger French et al. (Brookfield, Vt: Ashgate, 1998), 248–87.

43 Morbo gálico is the focus of Allen Shotwell's argument for a strain of medical humanism that sought to reemphasize the boundaries of surgery and physic. R. Allen Shotwell, "The Great Pox and the Surgeon's Role in the Sixteenth Century," *Journal of the History of Medicine and Allied Sciences* 72, no. 1 (2017): 21–33.

44 Andrés Alcázar, *Chirurgiae libri sex: in quibus multa antiquorum, et recentiorum sub obscura loca hactemus non declarata interpretantur* (Salamanca, 1575), 169–70; Fragoso, *Cirugia universal*, 255–255v; Calvo, *Cirugia uniuersal*, 1626, 567–69; León, *Practico de morbo gallico*, 2–4.

45 Jon Arrizabalaga, "The Changing Identity of the French Pox in Early Renaissance Castile," in *Between Text and Patient: the Medical Enterprise in Medieval & Early Modern Europe*, ed. Florence Eliza Glaze and Brian Nance, Micrologus' library 39 (Firenze: SISMEL, Edizioni del Galluzzo, 2011), 406–7; León, *Practico de morbo gallico*, 4; Calvo, *Cirugia uniuersal*, 1626, 564.

46 Arrizabalaga, Henderson, and French, *The Great Pox*, 266–9; William Eamon, "Cannibalism and Contagion: Framing Syphilis in Counter-Reformation Italy," *Early Science and Medicine* 3, no. 1 (1998): 1–31; Arrizabalaga, "The Changing Identity of the French Pox in Early Renaissance Castile," 403–5.

47 "[O]tras guerras civiles ha avido, donde los soldados han comido tan malos alimentos, y aun carnes de cavallos, y humanas, no sabiendolo ellos, y no llemos en ningun autor…a tener esta enfermedad." Calvo, *Cirugia uniuersal*, 1626, 568.
48 Calvo, 569.
49 See, for example Fragoso, *Cirugia universal*, 1592, fol. 255v. Unsurprisingly, Calvo disagrees with Fragoso Juan Calvo, *Primera y segunda parte de la cirugia uniuersal y particular del cuerpo humano* (Valencia, 1647), 56.
50 "Los remedios desta enfermedad, se diversifican segun las especies y variedad de los accidentes, cada uno de los quales requiere tambien su cura particular." Fragoso, *Cirugia universal*, 1596, 256.
51 Calvo, *Cirugia uniuersal*, 1626, 574.
52 Calvo, 579.
53 Hidalgo de Agüero, *Tesoro*, 12.

CONCLUSION

In the sixteenth century, surgeons throughout Europe worked to become learned in medical theory as well as skilled in surgical techniques. They innovated and improvised, kept abreast of what their colleagues were doing, and published voluminous surgical manuals, promoting their profession as one that encompassed both vernacular and learned traditions. The Spanish médico y cirujano, like his learned colleagues throughout Europe, embraced this new dual path of study and experience and then turned to challenging many traditions, refining old practices, and developing new ones.

The unique Spanish context in which these surgeons studied and worked had two important aspects, which were interconnected. The first was the rule of two strong monarchs, Charles V and Philip II, both of whom sought to exert control over many aspects of medical education and licensing. The second was the entrenched regionalism that these Habsburg monarchs were trying to overcome. Following the union of Fernando and Isabel in the fifteenth century, their descendants continued to rule a composite monarchy, made up of the separate territories of Castile, Aragon, Catalonia, Valencia, Navarre, and Portugal (after 1580). These territories each continued to maintain their own legislative bodies, law codes, rights, traditions, and cultures. These regional differences meant that the kings were unable to simply impose their will in matters, medical or otherwise. Charles V's efforts to expand the Protomedicato to these regions, for example, were resisted to varying degrees in most of them. Philip II's decrees introducing surgery into Castilian universities followed an example that already existed in Catalonia and Valencia. The monarchs were forced to continually negotiate with local authorities and customs, which enabled a range of different educational and licensing procedures. At the same time, the composite nature of the monarchy also meant that other territories under Spanish Hapsburg rule helped foster influence between Iberia, the Netherlands, and Italy, further enabling the circulation of people, texts, and ideas.

DOI: 10.4324/9781003291060-7

At the level of the practitioners themselves, this regionalism mattered little. As students, apprentices, and then practitioners, surgeons moved easily between different regions for study and work. We don't know what influenced these learned surgeons to attend university and then practice as surgeons. But once they did so, they turned to working in a wide range of settings, including at the royal court, in military service to various nobles, for municipalities, at universities, and in private practice, that allowed them to successfully reshape their profession. Their influence was likewise felt all across the peninsula as their texts were published (and republished) in many different cities from Seville to Barcelona, Valladolid to Valencia.

The refinement and expansion of knowledge these surgeons offered were grounded in familiarity with ancient and medieval authors and encouraged by the Renaissance humanist programs of linguistics, textual critique, and reinterpretation. Ultimately, an accumulation of personal experience and observational case studies inspired them all to become teachers, publishing texts that incorporated learning and personal experience. They wrote for students, for colleagues, and for posterity. Some, like Antonio Pérez and Juan Fragoso, wrote early in their careers, using their texts to establish themselves as learned experts. Most of them, however, wrote much later in their lives after they were established in the field and had garnered long experience. Those who wrote in Latin reflect the effort to raise the status of surgery to a learned field, separate from the specialized treatments of empirics and more equal with physic. Those who wrote in the vernacular also sought to raise the status of surgery, reaching out to a specific audience that was trained in surgery but not Latin.

Though most of these texts were written in the vernacular, they reflect the learned traditions of their time. Though some texts did contain a variety of recipes for unguents and poultices, they did not promise the revelation of secrets or proffer any general regimens in the manner of popular texts. Instead, they systematically discussed the conditions surgeons should treat, laying out various practices, along with extensive theory and frequent references to both predecessors and contemporaries. Their prose is often dense and unrelieved by images. Calling upon a long tradition of learned texts, Renaissance surgeons worked to effectively reshape surgery into a modern and progressive field. Though not all of the individuals included here have been remembered as reformers, many were highly innovative. But even those who disputed some new ideas and who advocated for more traditional approaches to healing were still part of the novel movement of educated surgeons who utilized medical theory and published their ideas.

Though many of these surgeons did not know each other personally, they were colleagues in an intellectual community whose members all sought to promote the best knowledge and practices possible. All of the surgeons considered here remained influential and well-respected through the next century as their texts continued to be republished, translated, and circulated. Their fame spread both geographically and temporally as their publications were carried not only across Europe but also out to the colonies, where they continued to be both argued with and expanded upon. Most of them had died by the turn of the seventeenth century, but their work and their reputations lived on in reprintings and incorporation into later texts until the end of the eighteenth. By the nineteenth century, even as their work had become eclipsed by newer innovations and new understandings of infection and disease, they remained well studied and tied together by historians looking back to the accomplishments of the earlier era.

It is not surprising that the most articulate and highly educated surgeons came to control the circulation of surgical knowledge in Spain, but it is worth noting that most of them chose not to restrict that knowledge to other university-educated practitioners. Instead, they enabled its continued circulation in the vernacular as well as in Latin. This effectively ensured that non-Latinate surgeons had access to current knowledge of anatomy, medical theory, and surgical practices. Given the frequent reprintings of these texts, it appears that interest in them continued steadily. Philip II has long been acknowledged as being innovative in bringing surgery into Castilian universities by creating new professorships and requiring its study. But we should also recognize the willingness of learned practitioners working outside of universities to spread rather than restrict current knowledge.

Renaissance surgeons set out a program of learning and practice that continued to reverberate through the next century. Seventeenth-century learned surgeons continued to study and compose texts in the same manner, engaging in many of the same intellectual debates as this previous generation. A recent study analyzes the texts of twenty-seven surgeons who published works over the course of the seventeenth century.[1] Two of the surgeons in this study overlap in that one, Bartolomé Hidalgo de Agüero and Andrés de León, as their texts were published just after the turn of the century. The remaining twenty-five mostly continued the Renaissance traditions of working to balance ancient and modern, theoretical and practical, and tradition and innovation.[2] Though these seventeenth-century surgeons, like those before them, wrote with a variety of interests and purposes, many of them also continued to revisit the same issues that had been debated in the previous century. Through much of the next century, for example, surgeons continued the debate on wet vs. dry healing begun by Hidalgo de Agüero and Fragoso. They also continued debates over the use of trepanation, the utility of applying particular medicaments, and the origins and causes of various diseases.[3] These later surgeons added discussion of additional illnesses, including measles, smallpox, and scrofula/phthisis, which were less explicitly addressed by sixteenth-century surgeons.[4]

The greatest change that occurred in this next century was in royal licensing. In 1603, Philip III reversed his father's policy and allowed *romancista* surgeons, with no formal university schooling, to earn their licenses through examination by the Protomedicato. In part, this likely reflected the change in rulers and advisors. It also likely reflected, as shown by Michele Clouse, the lack of students willing to complete the necessary studies in order to practice surgery, a lack also noted at some Italian universities in this era.[5] It is difficult to gauge the role played by these learned vernacular texts in this disinterest. On the one hand, they may well have provided sufficient knowledge of theory, which when combined with traditional practical training enabled surgeons to gain local licenses (if not royal ones). On the other hand, those who owned or read these texts may well have been already licensed practitioners seeking accessible (and up-to-date) reference works rather than students seeking textbooks. Philip III's decision to remove the educational prerequisites was likely influenced by other issues as well. One would have been the widespread plague epidemic at the turn of the century (1596–1602), which likely not only depleted the number of physicians and surgeons (along with the rest of the population) but also created a greater need for them.[6] In the immediate aftermath of the epidemic, the Castilian *Cortes* received petitions asking for the crown to make these changes in order to increase the number of surgeons available in rural areas.[7]

The removal of this requirement for royal licensing, however, did not mean the end of learned surgeons. The authors of surgical studies in the seventeenth century were a mix of university- and apprentice-trained. The earlier generation had earned their degrees without being required to, and many surgeons of the ensuing generations continued to do the same. The ongoing availability of the earlier Renaissance texts not only helped teach future generations but also may have inspired them to continue the work of both study and experiment.

Renaissance surgeons knew well what they wanted to accomplish. They set out to learn and experience, to test and innovate, to challenge and reshape the profession of surgery. They embraced the intellectual and technical movements of their era, writing and publishing learned vernacular texts in order to improve all surgical practice. In all these goals, they were immensely successful.

Notes

1 Lucía Aleixandre Porcar, "Las prácticas quirúrgicas en los libros de cirugía en castellano del siglo XVII" (Tesis doctoral, Universitat de València, 2020).
2 Francisco Salas Salgado, "Auctores y auctoritas en el 'Espejo de Chirurgia' de Antonio de Viana," *Ágora: Estudos Clássicos em Debate*, no. 18 (2016): 233–68.
3 Porcar, "Prácticas quirúrgicas," 543–4.
4 Porcar, 108–21.
5 Michele L Clouse, *Medicine, Government and Public Health in Philip II's Spain: Shared Interests, Competing Authorities* (Burlington, VT: Ashgate, 2011), 66; R. K French, "Berengario Da Carpi and the Use of Commentary in Anatomical Teaching," in *The Medical Renaissance of the Sixteenth Century*, ed. A. Wear, R. K. French, and Iain M. Lonie (New York: Cambridge University Press, 2009), 48.
6 Ruth MacKay, *Life in a Time of Pestilence: The Great Castilian Plague of 1596–1601* (New York: Cambridge University Press, 2019); Kristy Wilson Bowers, *Plague and Public Health in Early Modern Seville*, Rochester Studies in Medical History (Rochester, NY: University of Rochester Press, 2013).
7 Clouse, *Medicine, Government and Public Health in Philip II's Spain*, 108–9.

APPENDIX
Brief Biographies of Spanish Learned Surgeons

Andrés Alcázar (c.1490?–1585?)

Chirurgiae libri sex. In quibus multa antiquorum et recentiorum sub obscura loca hactenus non declarata interpretantur. Salamanca 1575.

De vulneribus capitis. Salamanca 1582.

Born in Guadalajara, possibly as early as 1490 or as late as 1510, Andrés Alcázar studied surgery under a local master, Antonio, whose daughter he later married. He also earned a medical degree from the University of Salamanca. He practiced for many years in Ávila, Segovia, and Guadalajara before becoming the first professor of surgery at the University of Salamanca in 1568. He remained there until his death, possibly in 1585.

Alcázar published one surgical text, *Chirurgiae libri sex* (1575), the first book of which, on head wounds, was republished as a freestanding text in 1582. The full text includes six books, the first of which is considered the most important for its detailed discussion of head wounds and their associated neurologic symptoms, as well as innovations in instruments for trepanation. The remaining books cover wounds to the nervous system, wounds of the thorax, wounds of the abdomen, morbo gálico, and plague (pestilential illness).

In the first book, Alcázar claims to have developed innovations in the construction of trepans as a young surgeon. He showed these to French surgeon Louis Delbourges, who accompanied King Francis I in his detainment in Spain (in 1525 during the Hapsburg-Valois Wars) and then took the design ideas back to France. Alcázar also accused Luis Lucena, a friend and colleague who had likewise seen these improved instruments, of sharing these ideas with others when he left for extended travels in Italy and France. Among those who later published on these innovations was Guido Guidi (Vidus Vidius) in a 1544 surgical text.

Francisco Arceo (d. 1580)

De recta curandorum vulnerum ratione. Antwerp 1574; Amsterdam 1658.

[London (English) 1588; Nuremberg (German) 1600, 1674, 1717; Paris (French) 1634; Holland (Dutch) 1667].

Francisco Arceo was born around 1493, most likely in Fregenal de la Sierra. Many of Arceo's biographical details are unclear. Early biographers assert that he studied medicine at Alcalá de Henares, but there are no documents to confirm this. In his work, he refers to a case at Guadalupe in 1516, so we can affirm he was practicing there at age 23 or 24, though whether he studied elsewhere first is unclear. His text is written in polished Latin, which would indicate university training, but here again, there is scholarly debate. Some have argued that while the content may be Arceo's, the writing style is closely aligned with that of his friend, the famous humanist Benito Arias Montano, who also wrote a preface to the text. Following his time at Guadalupe, Arceo spent his career in practice in towns between Badajoz and Seville, including the town of Llerena, where he worked for both municipal authorities and the local office of the Inquisition.

His 1574 Latin text is divided into two parts, one on surgery and the other principally on fevers. The first part includes a focus on head wounds: six chapters on cranial surgery, one on facial surgery, and eight on wounds of the chest, abdomen, and limbs. This is followed by four chapters on morbo gálico and a final chapter on treating clubfoot. The second part includes an antidotary and eight chapters on fevers.

Arceo generally advocated for less intervention in wounds when possible, much along the same lines as Bartolomé Hidalgo de Agüero. Arceo is also remembered for his healing balsam, which was not only included in the antidotaries of other contemporary surgeons but continued to appear in pharmacopeias into the 20th century. Among other innovations, Arceo developed an orthopedic boot to correct clubfoot in children, publishing this in a work that appeared the same year that Ambroise Paré also described the condition and a similar form of treatment.

Originally published in Antwerp by Plantin Press, Arceo's Latin text was later translated into English as *A Most Excellent and Compendious Method of Curing Woundes in the Head, and in Other Partes of the Body* in 1588 by John Read. Translations into French, German, and Dutch followed in the next century.

Juan Calvo (1535–99)

Primera y segunda parte de la cirugia universal y particular Sevilla 1580, 1598.

Madrid 1626, 1657, 1674; Perpigan 1636; Valencia 1599, 1646, 1647, 1690, 1703.

Poitiers 1614; Rouen 1656.

Libro muy util y provechoso de medicina, y cirugia, que trata de las cosas naturales, no naturales y preternaturales Barcelona 1591.

Libro de medicina y cirurgia que trata de las llagas en general y en particular Barcelona 1592.

Born in 1536, likely in Valencia, Juan Calvo studied medicine at the University of Valencia with Luis Collado and surgery in Zaragoza with Jerónimo Murillo. He spent some time teaching surgery in Montpellier before returning to Valencia, continuing his teaching career. It is not clear whether he was affiliated with the University of Valencia or taught privately (or some of each). His earliest publications (1592, 1596) list him as lecturer in surgery in the *city* of Valencia, but later editions (1626) list him as "lecturer in medicine at the University."

Calvo's full text, known as the *Primera y Segunda Parte*, was immensely popular and reprinted numerous times into the eighteenth century. The first part opens with a discussion of the theory of naturals, non-naturals, and preternaturals and then addresses two of the main issues faced by surgeons, tumors/swellings (apostemas) and wounds (llagas). For each of these, Calvo devotes one book to them in general and a second to particular types of each. In the second part, Calvo continues this format, addressing ulcers in general and then in particular. He completes the text with an antidotary.

Calvo's text was a very popular surgical manual, used in teaching and circulating widely as evidenced by the editions published in various cities throughout Spain. It also appears in many inventories in the New World.

Dionisio Daza Chacón (1503/1510–96)

La primera parte de la Cirujía que trata de los humores preternaturales Valladolid 1580.

Practica y teorica de cirugía en romance y latin Valladolid 1585,1595, 1605, 1609. Madrid 1619, 1626, 1678; Valencia 1650, 1673.

Segunda parte de la prática y theórica de Cirugía en romance, en latín que trata de todas las heridas Valladolid 1595.

Born in Valladolid, possibly in 1503 or 1510, Dionisio Daza Chacón's grandfather, father, and uncle were doctors. He studied first at the University of Valladolid and then completed medical studies at Salamanca by the early 1540s. Daza Chacón began his career in military service in Flanders in the service of Don Pedro de Guzmán and then moved up to serve Emperor Charles V himself. He went on to have a lengthy and active career in royal service, serving both in the military and in the households of various members of the royal family.

After the war in Flanders, Daza Chacón spent time attached to the households of various members of Charles's family, including his daughter María and son-in-law Prince Maximilian of Austria (later Maximillian II), his daughter Princess Juana (while she was in Portugal until her husband's untimely death), his grandson Don Carlos (son of Philip II), and his illegitimate son Don Juan de Austria. With the latter, Daza Chacón returned to military service, first within Spain at the Revolt of Alpujarras (1568–71) and subsequently in naval forces in the Mediterranean. In addition, Daza Chacón served six years as a surgeon at the Royal Hospital of Valladolid (Hospital Real de la Corte) and later served on the royal Protomedicato board of examiners for surgeons.

Daza Chacón composed his surgical treatises late in life, publishing when he had retired from active service. The texts address a standard suite of surgical issues including wounds, tumors/swellings, ulcers, and so forth. Yet Daza Chacón included many personal stories of cases he treated or witnessed, enlivening his work by adding his own views and experiences.

Daza Chacón's embrace of experiment and innovation is well-known. He recounts learning a gentler treatment for gunpowder wounds on the battlefield at the same time Ambroise Paré was testing his similar method. Among other things, he also describes gangrene, methods of amputation by ligating rather than cauterizing arteries, using a flap of skin to cover an amputated stump, using ligation to clip aneurisms, and treating nasal polyps.

Francisco Díaz (1527–90)

Compendio de chirugia en el cual se trata de todas las cosas tocantes a la teórica y prática della y de la anatomia del cuerpo humano Madrid 1575.

Tratado nuevamente impresso, de todas las enfermedades de los riñones, vexiga, y carnosidades de la verga, y urina, dividido en tres libros Madrid 1588, 1627, 1643.

Born in Alcalá de Henares in 1527, Francisco Díaz also studied at the university there, completing a bachelor of arts degree in 1548, and then continued his medical studies, traveling to Valencia to study anatomy and dissection with Luis Collado and Pedro Jimeno. Returning to Alcalá, he completed additional degrees, receiving a doctorate in medicine in 1555 and a master of philosophy in 1556.

Díaz initially applied for a position at the royal Hospital de la Corte in Valladolid but lost the position to Dionisio Daza Chacón. He moved instead to become a municipal surgeon in Burgos, where he remained until 1565. Married in 1550 to María de la Flor de Medrano, Díaz had five children. When a plague epidemic of 1564–5 took the lives of his wife and youngest daughter, he moved back to Alcalá where his siblings still lived. He soon married a second time, to Mariana de Vergara. The two had another six children, all born in Madrid after he succeeded in obtaining a position at the royal court in 1570.

Díaz published two texts, a compendium of surgery in 1575 and a treatise on urology in 1588. The surgical text is composed of four parts: anatomy, apostemas (tumors/swellings), heridas (fresh wounds), and ulcers (old wounds), to which is appended a final treatise on "four conditions necessary to understand and treat," which discusses hemorrhoids, hernia, impetigo (skin eruptions), and *nimphea* (a protrusion of tissue from female genitalia).

Díaz was the first to codify urology with his second text, which helped to establish this as a field of medicine. It is composed of three books: one on the kidneys, the second on the bladder, and the third on urinary stricture. In addition to pulling together anatomical and treatment information that had previously been scattered piecemeal in various older texts, Díaz developed new catheters and other instruments to treat various urogenital conditions.

Juan Fragoso (1530–97)

Catalogus simplicium medicamentorum Alcalá de Henares 1566.
Erotemas chirurgicos Madrid 1570, 1573.
Discurso de las cosas aromáticas Madrid 1572; Latin edition 1601.
De succedaneis medicamentis Mantua 1575; Madrid 1583; Sevilla 1632.
Cirugía universal Madrid 1581, 1586, 1596, 1627, 1643, 1666; Alcalá 1592, 1601, 1607, 1621; Zaragoza 1692.

Born in Toledo in 1530, Juan Fragoso studied at Alcalá de Henares, graduating with a medical degree in 1552. Fragoso then moved to Seville to practice. He became friends with Francisco Hernández and accompanied him on botanical excursions around the region. He moved to court in Madrid in 1570 where he served various members of the royal family for the next twenty years. He married and had at least three children who were born in Madrid.

Fragoso published three works on botany and one on surgery, which he continued to revise and expand in subsequent editions. The *Cirugía universal* includes two parts. Part one is composed of six books covering the standard topics of anatomy, tumors/swellings, fresh wounds, old wounds, fractures, and dislocations. The second part includes a gloss for the prior books and antidotary and three added treatises: a dismissal of Bartolomé Hidalgo de Agüero's treatise, a discussion of legal medicine, and a selection of Hippocrates' *Aphorisms*.

Fragoso was an adamant opponent of Bartolomé Hidalgo de Agüero but is remembered more for the popularity of both his botanical and surgical texts.

Bartolomé Hidalgo de Agüero (1531–97)

Avisos particulares de cirugía contra la común opinión Sevilla 1584.
Tesoro de la verdadero cirugia Sevilla 1604, Barcelona 1624, Valencia 1654.

Born in Seville in 1531, Bartolomé Hidalgo de Agüero was a true native son who never left the city. He studied at the university there and under his mentors Alonso Cuadra and Juan de la Cueva, replacing the latter as head surgeon at the Hospital del Cardenal after his death. Hidalgo de Agüero developed what he called the *vía particular*, an approach to wound healing that advocated as little intervention as possible, simply keeping wounds clean, dry, and lightly covered. His success in wound treatment earned him a high reputation throughout the city and inclusion in the artist Francisco Pacheco's *Libro de descripción de verdaderos Retratos, de ilustres y memorables varones*, a sort of portrait gallery of the illustrious men of Seville. Hidalgo de Agüero was married with three children.

The *Tesoro de la verdadero cirugia* (1604) was written late in Hidalgo de Agüero's life and published posthumously by his son-in-law, Francisco Ximénez Guillén. Hidalgo de Agüero advocated a "dry method" of wound healing, which eschewed interventions such as drainage tubes and tight, moist bandages. His methods were contested in his own time by Juan Fragoso and the dispute was continued by their students. Juan de Barrios, who studied with both Juan Calvo in Valencia and Juan Fragoso in Madrid included a treatise "against Doctor Hidalgo of Seville" in his *Verdadera medicina* (1607), while numerous students of Hidalgo de Agüero, including Juan de Sosa Sotomayor, Enrique Vaca de Alfaro, and Pedro López de León each published treatises defending the *vía particular*. As late as 1779, Hidalgo de Agüero was still being cited in a dissertation on surgical approaches for healing head wounds.

Andrés de León

Libro primero, de annathomia. Recopilaciones, y examen general de evacuaciones, annathomia y compostura del cuerpo humano, differencias y virtudes del anima, diffiniciones de medicina, con muchas cosas curiosas y provechosas de philosophia, y astrologia. Baeza, 1590.

Practico de morbo gallico, en el qual se contiene el origen conocimiento desta enfermedad, y el mejor modo de curarla Valladolid, 1605.

Tratados de medicina, cirugia, y anatomia Valladolid, 1605.

Most likely born in Granada, though the year is unknown, Andrés de León studied medicine in Seville and mentions working alongside Nicolas Monardes in two Seville hospitals, the Hospital de los Desamparados and the Hospital del Cardenal. From there he moved on to study and work at the Hospital General in Valencia and later the Hospital General in Zaragoza. By 1568, León was serving among the troops sent with Don Juan de Austria to quell the Revolt of the Alpujarras (1568–71). In 1579, he accompanied the Duke of Alcalá (Fernando Enriquez de Ribera) to bring the remains of Emperor Charles V and Empress Isabel from Yuste to the royal mausoleum built by Philip II at the royal residence of El Escorial. The following year, León accompanied troops with the Duke of Alba to Portugal in 1580 to claim the throne for Philip II. In 1588, he was Protomedicato de mar oceano and accompanied the Armada on its ill-fated attempt to invade England. León was among the fortunate who returned to Spain. In between these various military stints, León settled in Baeza, where he wrote and published the first of his works in 1590.

His 1590 text contains, as the title indicates, a wealth of anatomical, medical, and astrological information. His third text is virtually a reprint of this text with a new name and his treatise on morbo gálico added to the end. The four main books into which his text is divided are anatomy, medical astrology, surgery, and bleeding and purging.

Andrés de León was unique in incorporating a strong focus on astrology and the importance of understanding planetary influences when undertaking treatments, especially bleeding and purging.

Antonio Pérez

Suma y exámen de cirugía con breves esposiciones de algunas sentencias de Hipócrates y Galeno Madrid, 1568, 1604; Alcalá 1575, 1591;Valencia 1634 and 1649.

Tractado de peste y sus causas, señales y curacion Madrid, 1598.

All that is known of Antonio Pérez's background is that he was Portuguese and that he was at court by 1567 as noted in the royal license for publication of his text, *Summa y examen de cirugia*. This text is one of the earliest of the vernacular texts by a learned surgeon, though we have no clear record of Pérez's education.

Pérez was certainly serving in the forces under Don Juan de Austria at the Revolt of the Alpujarras (1568–71), along with Andrés de León and Dionisio Daza Chacón. He remained in the forces that went with Don Juan thereafter and, like Daza Chacón, was at the Battle of Lepanto in 1571. Continuing in the Mediterranean with the fleet afterward, he was captured and then ransomed in Tunis (1574). Upon his redemption, he traveled to the Netherlands to rejoin Don Juan where he remained for some years even after Don Juan's death in 1578. Returning to Spain, Pérez then served with the Duke of Alba in the 1580 Portuguese campaign, later returning to the Netherlands with the Conde de Fuentes. He returned to Spain by the end of the century, helping to oversee medical efforts there during the plague epidemic 1596–1600.

His surgical treatise is divided into five books: apostemas, recent wounds, old wounds, fractures and dislocations, and selections of Hippocrates' *Aphorisms* related to surgery.

BIBLIOGRAPHY

Primary sources

"1575 Codicilo Del Doctor Bernardino Daza Chacón, Médico y Padre Del Licenciado Dionisio Daza | Real Biblioteca | Investigadores." Accessed August 27, 2019. https://investigadoresrb.patrimonionacional.es/node/5714

Alcázar, Andrés. *Andreae Alcazaris Medici, ac Chirurgi Guadalaxarensis in amplissima Salmanticensi Academia Chirurgae facultatis primi Professoris Chirurgiae libri sex: in quibus multa antiquorum, et recentiorum sub obscura loca hactemus non declarata interpretantur*. Salamanca, 1575.

Alfaro, Enrique Vaca de. *Proposicion chirurgica i censura iudiciosa entre las dos vias curativas de heridas de cabeça comun i particular i elecion desta: con dos epistolas al fin, una de la naturaleza del tumor preternatural, i otra de la patria i origen de Auicena...* Sevilla: por Gabriel Ramos Vejarano, 1618.

Amusco, Juan Valverde de. *Historia de la composición del cuerpo humano*. Rome, 1556.

Arceo, Francisco. *De recta curandorum vulnerum ratione et aliis eius artis praeceptis libri II: eiusdem De febrium curandarum ratione*. ex officina Christophori Plantini, 1574.

Arceo de Fregenal, Francisco. *Método verdadero de curar las heridas y otros preceptos de este arte; Método de curar las fiebres*. Edited by Andrés Oyola Fabián and J. Cobos Bueno. Bibliotheca Montaniana 21. Huelva: Universidad de Huelva, 2009.

Aviñón, Juan de. *Sevillana Medicina: que trata el modo conservativo y curativo de los que habitan en... Sevilla (1545)*. Sevilla: Enrique Rasco, 1885.

Barrios, Juan de. *Verdadera medicina, cirugía y astrologia en tres libros dividida*. Fernando Balli, 1607.

Boschi, Ippolito. *De vulneribus a bellico fulmine illatis*, 1596.

Botallo, Leonardo. *De curandis vulneribus sclopettorum*. Rovillius, 1560.

Calvo, Juan. "Cirurgia de Guido de Cauliaco con la glosa de Falco: agora nueuamente corregida y emendada y muy añadida... con un tratado de los simples." Valencia: en casa de Pedro Patricio, 1596.

———. *Primera y segunda parte de la cirugia vniuersal y particular del cuerpo humano*. Madrid: Diego Flamenco, 1626.

———. *Primera y segunda parte de la cirugia vniuersal y particular del cuerpo humano*. Valencia, 1647.

———. *Primera y segunda parte de la cirugia vniuersal y particular del cuerpo humano*. Madrid, 1674.

———. *Segunda parte de la medicina y cirurgia, que trata de las vlceras en general y particular, y del Antidotario, en el qual se trata de la facultad de todos los medicame[n]tos assi simples como compuestos segun Gal. en el libro quarto y quinto de la facultad de los simples, con otros tratados.* Valencia, 1599.

Campbell, Eldridge and James Colton, trans. *The Surgery of Theodoric* New York: Appleton-Century-Crofts, Inc., 1955.

Carpi, Jacopo Berengario da. *Tractatus de fractura calve sive cranei.* Impressum per Hieronymum de Benedictis, 1518.

Celsus. *De Medicina.* Translated by W.G. Spencer. Perseus Digital Library. Accessed October 16, 2021. http://www.perseus.tufts.edu/hopper/text?doc=Perseus:text:1999.02.0142

Chauliac, Guy de. *Guy de Chauliac (A.D. 1363) on Wounds and Fractures.* Translated by W. A. Brennan. Chicago: Published by the Translator, 1923.

Croce, Giovanni Andrea dalla. *Cirurgia universale e perfetta di tutte le parti pertinenti all'ottimo chirurgo di nuovo posta in luce.* Giordano Ziletti, 1583.

Croce, Giovanni Andrea Della. *Chirurgiae Ioannis Andreae a Cruce, Veneti medici, libri septem.* Venetii, 1573.

Daza Chacón, Dionisio. *Practica y teorica de cirugia en romance y en latin.* Valladolid: en casa de Ana Velez, 1609.

———. *Pratica y teorica de cirugia en romance y en latin.* por Francisco Cipres, 1673.

———. "Relación verdadera de la herida de cabeza del serenísimo príncipe d. Carlos nuestro señor, de gloriosa memoria, la cual se acabó en fin de Julio del año 1562." In *Colección de Documentos inéditos para la historia de españa,* 18: 537–63. Madrid, 1842.

———. *Segunda parte de la pratica y teorica de cirugia en romance y en latin, que trata de todas las heridas en general, y en particular.* por la viuda de Alonso Martin, a costa de Domingo Gonçalez, 1626.

"Dichos de Medicos Sobre Si Ai Peste Este Ano de 1582," 1582. Seccion 13, siglo XVI, tomo 6, ff. 83–93. Archivo Municipal de Sevilla.

Díaz, Francisco. *Compendio de chirurgia: en el qual de trata de todas las cosas tocantes la theorica y pratica della.* Madrid, 1575.

———. *Tratado, nuevamente impresso, de todas las enfermedades de los riñones, vexiga, y carnosidades de la verga y urina: dividido en tres libros.* Madrid, 1588.

Early Modern Letters Online. "The Correspondence of Christophe Plantin." Accessed June 19, 2021. http://emlo-portal.bodleian.ox.ac.uk/collections/?catalogue=christophe-plantin

Falloppio, Gabriele. *De morbo gallico liber absolutissimus.* Venetiis: Apud Aegidium Regazolam, 1574.

Ferri, Alfonso, Giovanni Francesco Rota, and Leonardo Botallo. *De curandis vulneribus sclopetorum tractatus singulares.* Antverpiae: Ex officina Arnoldi Coninx, 1583.

Fragoso, Juan. *Catalogus simplicium medicamentorum.* Alcalá de Henares: P. Robles & J. Villanoua, 1566.

———. *Cirugia Universal … y mas otros tres tratados … el primero es, una summa de proposiciones contraciertos avisos de cirugia. El segundo, de las declaraciones acerca de diversas heridas y muertos. El tercero, de los aphorismos de hyppocrates tocantes a cirugia,* 1592.

———. *De succedaneis medicamentis liber denuo auctus…Ejusdem animadversiones, in quamplurima medicamenta composita, quoru[m] est usus in hispanicis officinis.* Madrid, 1575.

———. *Discurso de las cosas aromaticas, arboles y frutales y de otras muchas medicinas simples que se traen de la India Oriental y que siruen al vso de medicina.* Madrid: en casa de Francisco Sanchez, 1572.

———. *Erotemas chirurgicos en los que se enseña todo lo mas necessario del arte de cyrurgia…* por Pierres Cosin, a costa de Sebastian Yuañez, 1570.

Fragoso, Juan, and Francisco Díaz. *Cirugia vniuersal, aora nueuamenta añadida...: iten otros quatro tratados, el primero es vna suma de proposiciones contra auisos de cirugia, el segundo de las declaraciones acerca de diuersas heridas y muertes, el tercero, de los Aphorismos de Hipocrates tocantes a cirugia, el cuarto, de la naturaleza y calidades de los medicamentos simples; Iten vn tratado de todas las enfermedades de los riñones, vexiga y carnosidades de la verga y orina y de su cura...; por Francisco Diaz...* por la viuda de Alonso Martin, 1627.

Gago de Vadilla, Pedro. *Discursos de verdadera cirugia, y censura de ambas vias, y eleccion de la primera intencion curativa y unicion de las heridas*. Madrid, 1632.

Galen. *Method of Medicine*. Edited by Ian Johnston and G. H. R. Horsley. The Loeb Classical Library 516–18. Cambridge, MA: Harvard University Press, 2011.

Gerard, John. *The Herball Or Generall Historie of Plantes*. Norton, John, 1597.

Gersdorff, Hans von. *Feldbuch der Wundartzney*. Strasburg, 1517.

Hidalgo de Agüero, Bartolomé. *Thesoro de la verdadera cirugía y vía particular contra la común*. Sevilla: Francisco Pérez, 1604.

Hippocrates. *The Genuine Works of Hippocrates*. Translated by Frances Adams. Vol. II. New York: W. Wood and Company, 1886.

Hippocrates. *On Head Wounds*. Translated by Maury Hanson. Vol. I 4,1. Corpus Medicorum Graecorum. Berlin: Akademie Verlag, 1999.

Laguna, Andrés de. *Pedacio Dioscorides Anazarbeo, acerca de la materia medicinal y de los venenos mortiferos*, 1555.

León, Andrés de. *Libro primero de anatomía: recopilaciones y examen general*. Baeza: Juan Baptista de Montoya, 1590.

———. *Practico de morbo gallico, en el quel se contiene el origen y conocimiento della enfermedad, y el mejor modo de curarla*. Valladolid, 1605.

León, Pedro López de. *Pratica y teorica de las apostemas en general y particular: questiones y praticas de cirugia de heridas, llagas y otras cosas nuevas y particulares*. Sevilla: en la Oficina de Luys Estupiñan, 1628.

Leyva, Miguel Martinez de. *Remedios preservativos y curativos, para en tiempo de la peste, y otras curiosas experiencias divisos en dos cuercos ... compuesto por Miguel Martinez de Leyva...*, 1597.

López de León, Pedro. *Pratica y teorica de las apostemas en general y particular: questiones y praticas de cirugia de heridas, llagas y otras cosas nuevas y particulares*. Sevilla: en la Oficina de Luys Estupiñan, 1628.

Monardes, Nicolas. *Dos libros. El vno trata de todas las cosas que traen de nuestras Indias Occidentales, que siruen al vso de medicina, ... El otro libro, trata de los medicinas marauillosas que son contra todo veneno, la piedra Bezaar, y la yerua escuerçonera. Con la cura de los venenados. ... Agora nueuamente copuestos por el doctor Niculoso de Monardes medico de Seuilla*. Sevilla, 1565a.

Monardes, Nicolas. *Historia medicinal de las cosas que se traen de nuestras indias occidentales*. Sevilla, 1565b.

Muñoz, Miguel Eugenio. *Recopilación de las leyes, pragmaticas reales, decretos, y acuerdos del real tribunal del proto-medicato*. Valencia: En la Imprenta de la viuda de Antonio Bordazar, 1751.

Pacheco, Francisco. *Libro de descripcion de verdaderos retratos, de illustres y memorables varones*. Sevilla, 1599.

Paré, Ambroise. *Les oeuures d'Ambroise Paré: diuisees en vingt huict liures, auec les figures & portraicts, tant de l'anatomie que des instruments de chirurgie, & de plusieurs monstres: reueuës & augmentees par l'autheur*. Quatriesme edition: A Paris, 1575.

Pérez, Antonio. *Summa y examen de cirugia de lo mas necesario que en ella se contiene con breves exposiciones de algunas sentencias de Hipocrates y Galeno*. Madrid, 1568.

Rota, Giovanni Francesco. *De tormentariorum vulnerum natura, et curatione liber*. apud Anselmum Giaccarellum, 1555.

Sánchez de Oropesa, Francisco. *Discurso del doctor Francisco Sánchez de Oropesa para averiguar q[ue] mal de urina sea el q[ue] padece Diego Anriquez Leon su amigo i conpadre: en que incidentemente se tratan las cosas que parecieron dificultosas i de mas consideraciõ cerca de la essencia, causas, señales i cura de todos los males deste genero...* en casa de Iuan de Leon, 1594.
Spink, M. S. *Albucasis on Surgery and Instruments: A Definitive Edition of the Arabic Text with English Translation and Commentary*. G. L. Lewis, ed. Berkeley: University of California Press, 1973.
Tovar, Simón de. *De compositorum medicamentorum examine noua methodus* ... ex officina Christophori Plantini, 1586.
Vigo, Johannes de. *Practica in arte chirurgica*, 1516.

Secondary sources

Abadia Flores, Carolina. "La Comunidad Flamenca En Sevilla En El Siglo XVI." *Archivo Hispalense: Revista Histórica, Literaria y Artística* 282–4 (2010): 173–92.
Ackerknecht, Erwin H. "Early History of Legal Medicine." In *Legacies in Law and Medicine*, edited by Chester R. Burns, 249–71. New York: Science History Publications, 1977.
Agulló y Cobo, Mercedes. *Documentos sobre médicos españoles de los siglos XVI al XVIII*. Vol. XII. Cuadernos de Historia de La Medicina Española. Salamanca: Universidad de Salamanca, 1969.
Alvar, Antonio. *La universidad de Alcalá de Henares a principios del siglo XVI*. Alcalá de Henares: Universidad de Alcalá, 1996.
Alverny, Marie-Therese d'. "Translations and Translators." In *Renaissance and Renewal in the Twelfth Century*, edited by Robert Louis Benson, Giles Constable, Carol Dana Lanham, and Charles Homer Haskins. Cambridge, MA: Harvard University Press, 1982.
Amundsen, D. W. "Medicine and Surgery as Art or Craft: The Role of Schematic Literature in the Separation of Medicine and Surgery in the Late Middle Ages." *Transactions & Studies of the College of Physicians of Philadelphia*, 5, no. 1 (1979): 43–57.
Anderson, Robert R. "Alfonso X El Sabio and the Renaissance in Spain." *Hispania* 44, no. 3 (1961): 448. https://doi.org/10.2307/335406.
Anderson, T. "A Recently Discovered Mediaeval Bladder Stone from Norwich, with a Review of British Archaeological Bladder Stones and Documentary Evidence for Their Treatment." *BJU International* 88, no. 4 (2001): 351–4. https://doi.org/10.1046/j.1464-410X.2001.02298.x
Anteric, Ivana, Zeljana Basic, Katarina Vilovic, Kresimir Kolic, and Simun Andjelinovic. "Which Theory for the Origin of Syphilis Is True?" *The Journal of Sexual Medicine* 11, no. 12 (2014): 3112–18. https://doi.org/10.1111/jsm.12674.
Armelagos, George J., Molly K. Zuckerman, and Kristin N. Harper. "The Science Behind Pre-Columbian Evidence of Syphilis in Europe: Research by Documentary." *Evolutionary Anthropology: Issues, News, and Reviews* 21, no. 2 (2012): 50–7. https://doi.org/10.1002/evan.20340
Arráez Tolosa, Alfonso. "El paso de la epidemia de la peste atlántica de 1596–1602 por almansa." *Al-Basit* 63 (2018): 175–214.
Arrizabalaga, Jon. "Medical Causes of Death in Preindustrial Europe: Some Historiographical Considerations." *Journal of the History of Medicine and Allied Sciences* 54 (1999a): 241–60.
———. "Poor Relief in Counter-Reformation Castile: An Overview." In *Health Care and Poor Relief in Counter-Reformation Europe*, edited by Ole Peter Grell, Andrew Cunningham, and Jon Arrizabalaga, 151–76. New York: Routledge, 1999b.

———. "Problematizing Retrospective Diagnosis in the History of Disease." *Asclepio: Revista de Historia de La Medicina y de La Ciencia* 54, no. 1 (2002): 51–70.

———. "Spanish Medical Students' Peregrinato to Italian Universities in the Renaissance." In *Centres of Medical Excellence? Medical Travel and Education in Europe 1500–1789*, edited by Ole Peter Grell, Andrew Cunningham, and Jon Arrizabalaga, 93–126. Burlington, VT: Ashgate, 2010.

———. "The Changing Identity of the French Pox in Early Renaissance Castile." In *Between Text and Patient: The Medical Enterprise in Medieval & Early Modern Europe*, edited by Florence Eliza Glaze and Brian Nance, 397–417. Micrologus' library 39. Firenze: SISMEL, Edizioni del Galluzzo, 2011.

Arrizabalaga, Jon, John Henderson, and R. K. French. *The Great Pox: The French Disease in Renaissance Europe*. New Haven, CT: Yale University Press, 1997.

Barona, Josep Lluís. *Sobre medicina y filosofía natural en el renacimiento*. Valencia: Seminari d'Estudis sobre la Ciencia, 1993.

Barona, Josep Lluís, and Xavier Gómez i Font. *La correspondencia de Carolus Clusius con los científicos españoles*. València: Seminari d'Estudis Sobre la Ciència, 1998.

Barrera-Osorio, Antonio. *Experiencing Nature: The Spanish American Empire and the Early Scientific Revolution*. Austin, TX: University of Texas Press, 2006.

Bartolini, Donatella. "On the Borders: Surgeons and Their Activities in the Venetian State (1540–1640)." *Medical History* 59, no. 01 (2015): 83–100. https://doi.org/10.1017/mdh.2014.72

Beaujouan, Guy. "La medicina y la cirugía en el monasterio de Guadalupe." *Asclepio: Revista de Historia de La Medicina y de La Ciencia* 17 (1965): 155–70.

Beier, Lucinda McCray. "Seventeenth-Century English Surgery: The Casebook of Joseph Binns." In *Medical Theory, Surgical Practice*, 48–84. New York: Routledge, 1992.

Beltrán de Heredia y Onís, José María. "Dionisio Daza Chacón, cirujano del Renacimiento: su aportación al tratamiento de las heridas: lección inaugural del curso 1971–1972/de la Universidad de Valladolid," 1971. http://uvadoc.uva.es:80/handle/10324/4126

Bennett, H. S. "Science and Information in English Writings of the Fifteenth Century." *The Modern Language Review* 39, no. 1 (1944): 1. https://doi.org/10.2307/3716452

Benson, Robert Louis, Giles Constable, Carol Dana Lanham, and Charles Homer Haskins, eds. *Renaissance and Renewal in the Twelfth Century*. Cambridge, MA: Harvard University Press, 1982.

Berco, Cristian. *From Body to Community: Venereal Disease and Society in Baroque Spain*. Toronto: University of Toronto Press, 2016.

Bertoloni Meli, Domenico, and Cynthia Klestinec. "Renaissance Surgery Between Learning and Craft." *Journal of the History of Medicine and Allied Sciences* 72, no. 1 (2017): 1–5. https://doi.org/10.1093/jhmas/jrw043

Biersack, Martin. "The Adoption of Humanism in Catholic Spain (1470–1520)." *Reformation & Renaissance Review* 21, no. 1 (2019): 27–46. https://doi.org/10.1080/14622459.2019.1568371

Biraben, Jean-Noël. "Diseases in Europe: Equilibrium and Breakdown of the Pathocenosis." In *Western Medical Thought from Antiquity to the Middle Ages*, edited by Mirko D. Grmek and Bernardino Fantini, translated by Antony Shugaar, 319–53. Cambridge, MA: Harvard University Press, 1998.

Blanco Pérez, José Ignacio. *Humanistas Médicos en el Renacimiento vallisoletano*. Burgos: Universidad de Burgos, 1999.

Boucher, Caroline, and Geneviève Dumas. "Traductions et compilations médicales: Une coïncidence obligée?" *Early Science and Medicine* 17, no. 3 (2012): 273–308. https://doi.org/10.1163/157338212X645094

Bouley, Bradford. *Pious Postmortems: Anatomy, Sanctity, and the Catholic Church in Early Modern Europe*. Philadelphia: University of Pennsylvania Press, 2017.

Bowers, Barbara S., ed. *The Medieval Hospital and Medical Practice*. AVISTA Studies in the History of Medieval Technology, Science and Art, v. 3. Burlington, VT: Ashgate, 2007.

Bowers, Kristy Wilson. *Plague and Public Health in Early Modern Seville*. Rochester Studies in Medical History. Rochester, NY: University of Rochester Press, 2013.

———. "Tradition and Innovation in Spanish Medicine: Bartolomé Hidalgo de Agüero and the Vía Particular." *Sixteenth Century Journal* XLI, no. I (2010): 29–47.

Boxer, C. R. *Two Pioneers of Tropical Medicine: Garcia d'Orta and Nicolas Monardes*. Diamante, 14. London: Hispanic & Luso-Brazilian Councils, 1963.

Brockbank, William. "The Man Who Was Vidius." *Annals of The Royal College of Surgeons of England* 19, no. 5 (1956): 269–95.

Brockliss, Laurence, and Colin Jones. *The Medical World of Early Modern France*. New York: Oxford University Press, 1997.

Brown, Ted. "Word Wars: The Debate over the Use of the Vernacular in Medical Writings of the English Renaissance." *Texas Studies in Literature and Language* 37, no. 1 (1995): 98.

Burke, Peter. "Translations into Latin in Early Modern Europe." In *Cultural Translation in Early Modern Europe*, edited by Peter Burke and R. Po-Chia Hsia, 65–80. Cambridge: Cambridge University Press, 2007. https://doi.org/10.1017/CBO9780511497193.005

Burnett, Charles. "The Coherence of the Arabic-Latin Translation Program in Toledo in the Twelfth Century." *Science in Context* 14, no. 1–2 (2001): 249–88.

———. "The Institutional Context of Arabic-Latin Translations of the Middle Ages: A Reassessment of the 'School of Toledo.'" In *Vocabulary of Teaching and Research Between Middle Ages and Renaissance*, edited by Olga Weijers, 8: 214–35. Turnhout: Brepols Publishers, 1995. https://doi.org/10.1484/M.CIVI-EB.4.00129

Burns, Robert Ignatius, ed. *Emperor of Culture: Alfonso X the Learned of Castile and His Thirteenth-Century Renaissance*. Philadelphia: University of Pennsylvania Press, 1990.

Burns, S.J., Robert I., ed. "Stupor Mundi: Alfonso X of Castile, the Learned." In *Emperor of Culture: Alfonso X the Learned of Castile and His Thirteenth-Century Renaissance*, 1–13. Philadelphia: University of Pennsylvania Press, 1990.

Bylebyl, Jerome J. "The School of Padua: Humanistic Medicine in the Sixteenth Century." In *Health, Medicine and Mortality in the Sixteenth Century*, edited by Charles Webster, 335–70. New York: Cambridge University Press, 1979.

Byrne, Susan. *Ficino in Spain*. Toronto Iberic. Toronto: University of Toronto Press, 2015.

Campos Díez, María Soledad. "El Protomedicato en la administración central de la Monarquía Hispánica." *Dynamis: Acta Hispanica ad Medicinae Scientiarumque Historiam Illustrandam* 16, no. 0 (1996): 43–58.

———. *El Real Tribunal del Protomedicato Castellano, siglos XIV–XIX*. Cuenca: Ediciones de la Universidad de Castilla-La Mancha, 1999.

Campos y Fernandez de Sevilla, Francisco Javier, ed. *La ciencia en el Monasterio del Escorial*. Madrid: Ediciones Escurialenses, 1992.

Cano Pavón, José Manuel. *La ciencia En Sevilla (Siglos XVI–XX)*. Serie Filosofía y Letras, núm. 157. Sevilla: Universidad de Sevilla, 1993.

Carmona García, Juan Ignacio. *El sistema de hospitalidad pública en la Sevilla del antiguo régimen*. Sevilla: Excma. Diputación Provincial de Sevilla, 1979.

———. *Enfermedad y sociedad en los primeros tiempos modernos*. Sevilla: Secretariado de Publicaciones de la Universidad de Sevilla, 2005.

Carré, Antònia. "The Medieval Catalan Translations of Hippocrates' 'Aphorisms' | Ciència. Cat." Translated by Andrew Stacey. Ciència.cat: La ciència en la cultura catalana a l'Edat Mitjana i el Renaixement, September 29, 2017. https://sciencia.cat/temes/medieval-catalan-translations-hippocrates-aphorisms

Carreras Panchón, Antonio. "Dos testimonios sobre la epidemia de peste de 1599 en Valladolid." *Asclepio: Revista de Historia de La Medicina y de La Ciencia* 25 (1973): 351–7.

———. "Juan Fragoso En La Historia de La Medicina Legal." In *La Obra de Juan de Villarreal y Otros Estudios Historico-Medicos*. Salamanca: Universidad de Salamanca, 1978a.

———. *La Obra de Juan de Villarreal y Otros Estudios Historico-Medicos*. Cuadernos de Historia de La Medicina Española. Monografias 33. Salamanca: Ediciones Universidad de Salamanca, 1978b.

Casal, Marta Cacho. "The 'True Likenesses' in Francisco Pacheco's Libro de Retratos: Francisco Pacheco's Libro de Retratos." *Renaissance Studies* 24, no. 3 (2010): 381–406. https://doi.org/10.1111/j.1477-4658.2009.00599.x

Caso Amador, Rafael. "Bibliografía Sobre El Humanista Benito Arias Montano (1832–2005)." *Etiópicas: Revista de Letras Renacentistas* 1 (2005–4): 271–304.

Castiglioni, Arturo. *A History of Medicine*. Translated by E. B. Krumbhaar. 2nd ed. New York: Knopf, 1947.

Catalá, José Sala. *España en los siglos XV y XVI*. AKAL Historia de la ciencia y de la técnica, 14. Ediciones AKAL, 1992.

Cavallo, Sandra. *Artisans of the Body in Early Modern Italy: Identities, Families and Masculinities*. New York: Manchester University Press, 2007.

———. "Early Vernacular Medical Advice Books and Their Popular Appeal in Early Modern Italy." *Nuncius* 36, no. 2 (2021): 264–303. https://doi.org/10.1163/18253911-03602003

Chabrán, Rafael. "Dr. Francisco Hernández and Denmark: The Presence of The Mexican Treasury in the Work of Ole Worm. An Introduction." *The Colorado Review of Hispanic Studies* 7 (2009): 169–83.

———. "The Classical Tradition in Renaissance Spain and New Trends in Philology, Medicine, and Materia Medica." In *Searching for the Secrets of Nature: The Life and Works of Dr. Francisco Hernández*, edited by Simon Varey and Rafael Chabrán, 21–32. Stanford, CA: Stanford University Press, 2000.

Chinchilla, Anastasio. *Anales Históricos de la Medicina en General y Biográfico-Bibliográficos de la Española en Particular (1841–1846)*. 4 vols. http://147.156.5.138/Morejon_Chinchilla/

Clair, Colin. *Christopher Plantin*. London: Cassell & Company, 1960. https://www.biblio.com/book/christopher-plantin-clair-colin/d/1388111646

Clouse, Michele L. *Medicine, Government and Public Health in Philip II's Spain: Shared Interests, Competing Authorities*. Burlington, VT: Ashgate, 2011.

Cobos, José Miguel, and José Ramón Vallejo. "Francisco Arceo, médico del Santo Oficio de la Inquisición de Llerena." *Inquisición: XV Jornadas de Historia en Llerena* (2014): 299–310.

Cobos-Bueno, José M, Andrés Oyola Fabián, and Juan Fernando García Ávila. "El bálsamo de Francisco Arceo de Fregenal." *Llull* 33 (2010): 241–68.

Cohn, Samuel. *Cultures of Plague: Medical Thinking at the End of the Renaissance*. Oxford: Oxford University Press, 2011.

Comas, Juan. "Influencia de La Farmacopea y Terapeutica Indigenas de Nueva Espana En La Obra de Juan de Barrios." *Anales de Antropologia* 8 (1971): 125–50.

Conde Parrado, Pedro. "Ciencia y Cultura Clásica en la Cirugía Españolas Renacentista: el vallisoletano Dionisio Daza Chacón." *Argaya: revista provincial de cultura* 14 (1998): 13–20. http://uvadoc.uva.es:80/handle/10324/3590

———. "«Por el orden de Celso»: aspectos de la influencia del 'De medicina' en la Cirugía Europea del Renacimiento." *Dynamis: Acta Hispanica ad Medicinae Scientiarumque Historiam Illustrandam* 28(2008): 217–42.

Conforti, Maria. "Surgery, Medicine and Natural Philosophy in the Library of Marco Aurelio Severino (1580–1656)." *Bruniana & Campanelliana* 10, no. 2 (2004): 283–98.

Cook, Alexandra Parma, and Noble David Cook. *The Plague Files: Crisis Management in Sixteenth-Century Seville*. Baton Rouge: Louisiana State University Press, 2009.

Corbella Corbella, Jacinto. "El crecimiento del saber medico legal en España en el siglo XVI." *Asclepio: Revista de Historia de La Medicina y de La Ciencia* 30–31 (89 1978–9): 323–37.

Crawford, Catherine. "Legalizing Medicine: Early Modern Legal Systems and the Growth of Medico-Legal Knowledge." In *Legal Medicine in History*, edited by Michael Clark and Catherine Crawford. New York: Cambridge University Press, 1994.

Cunningham, Andrew. "Identifying Disease in the Past: Cutting the Gordian Knot." *Asclepio* 54, no. 1 (2002): 13–34. https://doi.org/10.3989/asclepio.2002.v54.i1.133

Dandelet, Thomas James. *Spanish Rome, 1500–1700*. New Haven, CT: Yale University Press, 2008.

Daston, Lorraine, and Elizabeth Lunbeck, eds. *Histories of Scientific Observation*. Chicago, IL: University of Chicago Press, 2011a.

———. "Observation Observed." In *Histories of Scientific Observation*, edited by Lorraine Daston and Elizabeth Lunbeck, 1–9. Chicago, IL: University of Chicago Press, 2011b.

Dávila, Joaquín Herrera, and José Joaquín Jadraque Sánchez. "El 'Tractatus de curatione' – 1606 – de Juan Sosa Sotomayor." *Archivo Hispalense: Revista histórica, literaria y artística* 91, no. 276 (2008): 93–129.

Debus, Allen G. *Man and Nature in the Renaissance*. Cambridge: Cambridge University Press, 1995.

——— "Paracelsus and the Delayed Scientific Revolution in Spain." In *Reading the Book of Nature: The Other Side of the Scientific Revolution*, edited by Allen G. Debus and Michael Thomson Walton, 147–61. Sixteenth Century Essays & Studies, v. 41. Kirksville, MO: Sixteenth Century Journal Publishers, 1998.

Delgado Jara, Inmaculada, and Rosa M. Herrera García. "Humanidades y humanistas en la Universidad de Salamanca del siglo XV." In *Salamanca y su universidad en el primer Renacimiento: Siglo XV*, 37. Miscelanea Alfonso IX. Salamanca: Universidad de Salamanca, 2010.

Demaitre, Luke E. *Medieval Medicine: The Art of Healing, from Head to Toe*. Santa Barbara, CA: Praeger, 2013.

De Renzi, Silvia. "Medical expertise, bodies, and the law in early modern courts." *Isis* 98, no. 2 (2007): 315–22. https://doi.org/10.1086/518191

De Renzi, Silvia, Marco Bresadola, and Maria Conforti, eds. *Pathology in Practice: Diseases and Dissections in Early Modern Europe*. New York: Routledge, 2019.

De Vos, Paula. "Pharmacopoeias and the Textual Tradition in Galenic Pharmacy." In *Drugs on the Page: Pharmacopoeias and Healing Knowledge in the Early Modern Atlantic World*, edited by Matthew James Crawford and Joseph M. Gabriel, 19–44. Pittsburgh, PA: University of Pittsburgh Press, 2019.

———. "The Science of Spices: Empiricism and Economic Botany in the Early Spanish Empire." *Journal of World History* 17, no. 4 (2006): 399–427. https://doi.org/10.1353/jwh.2006.0054

DeVries, Kelly R. "Military Surgical Practice and the Advent of Gunpowder Weaponry." *Canadian Bulletin of Medical History* 7, no. 2 (1990): 131–46. https://doi.org/10.3138/cbmh.7.2.131

Dingwall, Helen M. *Physicians, Surgeons and Apothecaries: Medicine in Seventeenth-Century Edinburgh*. East Linton: Tuckwell Press, 1995.

Domínguez Ortiz, Antonio. *The Golden Age of Spain, 1516–1659*. Translated by James Casey. History of Spain. New York: Basic Books, 1971.

Dowling, Kamilah A., and James Tait Goodrich. "Two Cases of 16th Century Head Injuries Managed in Royal European Families." *Neurosurgical Focus* 41, no. 1 (2016): E2. https://doi.org/10.3171/2016.4.FOCUS15119

Durling, Richard J. "A Chronological Census of Renaissance Editions and Translations of Galen." *Journal of the Warburg and Courtauld Institutes* 24, no. 3/4 (1961): 230. https://doi.org/10.2307/750797

Eamon, William. "Cannibalism and Contagion: Framing Syphilis in Counter-Reformation Italy." *Early Science and Medicine* 3, no. 1 (1998): 1–31.

———. *Science and the Secrets of Nature: Books of Secrets in Medieval and Early Modern Culture*. Princeton, NJ: Princeton University Press, 1994.

———. "The Charlatan's Trial. An Italian Surgeon in the Court of King Phillip II, 1576–1577." *Cronos. Cuadernos Valencianos de Historia de La Medicina y de La Ciencia* 8 (2000): 3–30.

———. "The Legend of Ambroise Paré and the 'Liberation' of Surgery." *William Eamon* (blog). Accessed July 11, 2020. https://williameamon.com/?p=297

———. *The Professor of Secrets: Mystery, Medicine, and Alchemy in Renaissance Italy*. Washington, DC: National Geographic, 2010.

Edwards, John. *The Spain of the Catholic Monarchs, 1474–1520*. Malden, MA: Blackwell Publishers, 2000.

Egmond, Florike, P. G. Hoftijzer, and Robert Paul Willem Visser, eds. *Carolus Clusius: Towards a Cultural History of a Renaissance Naturalist*. History of Science and Scholarship in the Netherlands, v. 8. Amsterdam: Koninklijke Nederlandse Akademie van Wetenschappen, 2007.

Eisenberg, Daniel. "La Biblioteca de Cervantes." In *Studia in honorem prof. M. de Riquer*, II:271–328. Barcelona: Quaderns Crema, 1986.

Engelmann, Lukas, John Henderson, and Christos Lynteris, eds. *Plague and the City*. New York: Routledge, 2019.

Feingold, Mordechai, and Víctor Navarro Brotons, eds. *Universities and Science in the Early Modern Period*. Archimedes, v. 12. Dordrecht: Springer, 2006.

Fernández Álvarez, Manuel, Luis Enrique Rodríguez-San Pedro Bezares, and Julián Alvarez Villar. *The University of Salamanca: Eight Centuries of Scholarship*. Salamanca: Ediciones Universidad de Salamanca, 1992.

Fernández Doctor, Asunción. "El control de las profesiones sanitarias en Aragón: el Protomedicato y los Colegios." *Dynamis: Acta Hispanica ad Medicinae Scientiarumque Historiam Illustrandam* 16 (1996): 173–85.

———. "Médicos y cirujanos de zaragoza en la edad moderna. Su número y estructura sociofamiliar." *Dynamis: Acta Hispanica ad Medicinae Scientiarumque Historiam Illustrandam* 17 (1997): 141–64.

Forrester, John M. "The Marvellous Network and the History of Enquiry into Its Function." *Journal of the History of Medicine and Allied Sciences* 57, no. 2 (2002): 198–217.

French, R. K. "Berengario Da Carpi and the Use of Commentary in Anatomical Teaching." In *The Medical Renaissance of the Sixteenth Century*, edited by A. Wear, R. K. French, and Iain M. Lonie, 42–74. New York: Cambridge University Press, 2009.

French, Roger, and Jon Arrizabalaga. "Coping with the French Disease: University Practitioners' Strategies and Tactics in the Transition from the Fifteenth to the Sixteenth Century." In *Medicine from the Black Death to the French Disease*, edited by Roger French, Jon Arrizabalaga, Andrew Cunningham, and Luis Garcia-Ballester, 248–87. Brookfield, VT: Ashgate, 1998.

French, Roger, Jon Arrizabalaga, Andrew Cunningham, and Luis Garcia-Ballester, eds. *Medicine from the Black Death to the French Disease*. Brookfield, VT: Ashgate, 1998.

Fresquet Febrer, José L. "El interés del estudio de la cirugía en la Monarquía Hispánica (s. XVI)." In *Más allá de la Leyenda Negra: España y la revolución científica = Beyond the Black Legend; Spain and the Scientific Revolution*, edited by Víctor Navarro Brotons and William Eamon, 295–306. Valencia: Universidad de València, Inst. de Historia de la Ciencia y Documentación López Piñero, 2007.

Fresquet Febrer, Jose Luis, ed. *Juan Calvo y la cirugía valenciana del siglo xvi: Simposio 2002 sobre la historia de la medicina*. València: Editorial Denes, 2002a.

Fresquet Febrer, Jose Luis. "La diversidad de mentalidades en la 'Cirugia' (1580) de Juan Calvo, a través del estudio de sus referencias." In *Estudios sobre la medicina y ciencia valencianas (siglos XVI–XIX)*, edited by M. José Báguena Cervellera, José Luis Barona Vilar, José Luis Fresquet Febrer, M. Luz López Terrada, Juan Antonio Micó Navarro, and Vicente Luis Salavert Fabiana, 71–89. Valencia: Universidad de Valencia, 1985.

———. "La fundación y desarrollo de los jardines botánicos." In *Felipe II, la Ciencia y la Técnica*, edited by Enrique Martínez Ruiz, 28. Madrid: Editorial Actas, 1999.

———. "La práctica médica en los textos quirúrgicos españoles en el siglo XVIII." *Dynamis: Acta Hispanica ad Medicinae Scientiarumque Historiam Illustrandam* 22 (2002b): 251–77.

———. "Materia médica americana en textos médicos espanoles del siglo XVI." *Cirugía y Cirujanos* 63, no. 2 (April 1995).

Fresquet Febrer, José Luis, María de la Luz López Terrada, and Carla Pilar Aguirre Marco. *La historia de la Medicina española de Hernández Morejón y de Chinchilla*. Valencia: Instituto de Historia de la Ciencia y Documentación López Piñero, 2007. http://147.156.5.138/Morejon_Chinchilla/

Front, Dov. "The Expurgation of Medical Books in Sixteenth-Century Spain." *Bulletin of the History of Medicine* 75, no. 2 (2001): 290–6. https://doi.org/10.1353/bhm.2001.0067.

Furdell, Elizabeth Lane, ed. *Textual Healing: Essays on Medieval and Early Modern Medicine*. Boston: Brill, 2005.

Gallardo, Bartolomé José. *Ensayo de una biblioteca española de libros raros y curiosos*. Vol. III. Madrid: Manuel Tello, 1888.

Gallent Marco, Mercedes. "El colegio de barberos y cirujanos de Valencia: aportación documental." *Saitabi*, 1993, No. 43: 147–55, 1993. https://roderic.uv.es/handle/10550/27064

———. "Precedentes medievales de la medicina legal: la 'dessospitació' en el reino de Valencia." *Saitabi* 50 (2000): 11–28.

García, Angelina. "Tres Bibliotecas de Medicos Valencianos Renacentistas." *Asclepio: Revista de Historia de La Medicina y de La Ciencia* 26–7 (75 1974): 527–46.

García Ballester, Luis, *La búsqueda de la salud: sanadores y enfermos en la españa medieval*. Historia, Ciencia y Sociedad 321. Barcelona: Ediciones Península, 2001.

———. "La cirugía en la Valencia del siglo XV. El privilegio de desecar cadaveres en 1477." *Cuadernos de Historia de La Medicina Espanola* 7 (1967): 155–76.

———. "Medical Science and Medical Teachings at the University of Salamanca in the 15th Century." In *Universities and Science in the Early Modern Period*, edited by Mordechai Feingold and Víctor Navarro Brotons, 36–64. Archimedes, v. 12. Dordrecht: Springer, 2006.

García Ballester, Luis, ed. *Historia de la ciencia y de la técnica en la Corona de Castilla*. Valladolid: Junta de Castilla y León, Consejería de Educación y Cultura, 2002.

García Ballester, Luis, Jon Arrizabalaga, and Fernando Salmón. "A propósito de las relaciones intelectuales entre la Corona de Aragón e Italia (1470–1520): Los estudiantes de medicina valencianos en los estudios generales de Siena, Pisa, Ferrara y Padua." *Dynamis: Acta Hispanica ad Medicinae Scientiarumque Historiam Illustrandam* 9 (1989): 117–47.

García Ballester, Luis, Roger French, Jon Arrizabalaga, and Andrew Cunningham, eds. *Practical Medicine from Salerno to the Black Death*. Cambridge: Cambridge University Press, 1994.

García Ballester, Luis, M. R. McVaugh, and Agustín Rubio. *Medical Licensing and Learning in Fourteenth-Century Valencia*. Transactions of the American Philosophical Society, v. 79, pt. 6. Philadelphia: American Philosophical Society, 1989.

García Ballester, Luis. "Academicism versus Empiricism in Practical Medicine in Sixteenth-Century Spain with Regard to Morisco Practitioners." In *The Medical Renaissance of the*

Sixteenth Century, edited by A. Wear, R. K. French, and Iain M. Lonie, 246–70. New York: Cambridge University Press, 2009.
García, Sebastián. "Medicina y Cirugía En Los Reales Hospitales de Guadalupe." *Revista de Estudios Extremeños* 59, no. 1 (2003): 11–77.
Gentilcore, David. "'All That Pertains to Medicine': Protomedici and Protomedicati in Early Modern Italy." *Medical History* 38, no. 2 (1994): 121–42. https://doi.org/10.1017/S0025727300059068
———. *Healers and Healing in Early Modern Italy*. New York: St. Martin's Press, 1998.
Getz, F.M. "Charity, Translation, and the Language of Medical Learning in Medieval England." *Bulletin of the History of Medicine* 64, no. 1 (March 1990): 1–17.
Glaze, Florence Eliza, and Brian Nance, eds. *Between Text and Patient: The Medical Enterprise in Medieval & Early Modern Europe*. Micrologus' library 39. Firenze: SISMEL, Edizioni del Galluzzo, 2011.
Gómez Ochoa, Fidel, and Daniel Macías Fernández, eds. *El combatiente a lo largo de la historia: imaginario, percepción, representación*. Santander: Universidad de Cantabria, 2012.
Gonzalez Muñoz, María del Carmen. "Epidemias y Enfermedades En Talavera de La Reina (SS. XVI y XVII)." *Hispania* 126 (1974): 149–68.
González Sánchez, Carlos Alberto. *New World Literacy: Writing and Culture across the Atlantic, 1500–1700*. Translated by Tristán Platt and Bethany Aram. Lewisburg PA: Bucknell University Press, 2011.
———, ed. *Sevilla, Felipe II y La Monarquía Hispánica*. Sevilla: Ayuntamiento de Sevilla, 1999.
González-Darder, José M. *Trepanation, Trephining and Craniotomy: History and Stories*. Springer Nature, 2019. https://doi.org/10.1007/978-3-030-22212-3.
Goodman, David C. *Power and Penury: Government, Technology, and Science in Philip II's Spain*. New York: Cambridge University Press, 1988.
Granjel, Luis S. *Cirugía Española Del Renacimiento*. Salamanca: Universidad de Salamanca, 1968.
———. *La Medicina Española Renacentista*. Historia General de La Medicina Española, II. Salamanca: Universidad de Salamanca, 1980.
———. "La Obra de Andrés Alcázar." *Clínica Y Laboratorio* LXVII, no. 395 (1959): 154–60.
Green, Monica. "Crafting a (Written) Science of Surgery: The First European Surgical Texts." *REMEDIA* (blog), October 13, 2015. https://remedianetwork.net/2015/10/13/crafting-a-written-science-of-surgery-the-first-european-surgical-texts/
Green, Monica H., and Brian Long. "Ego Constantinus Africanus Montis Cassinensis Monacus." *Constantinus Africanus* (blog), n.d. https://constantinusafricanus.com/
Green, Monica Helen, ed. *The Trotula: A Medieval Compendium of Women's Medicine*. Philadelphia: University of Pennsylvania Press, 2001.
Grell, Ole Peter, Andrew Cunningham, and Jon Arrizabalaga, eds. *Centres of Medical Excellence? Medical Travel and Education in Europe 1500–1789*. Aldershot: Ashgate, 2010.
———, eds. *Health Care and Poor Relief in Counter-Reformation Europe*. New York: Routledge, 1999.
Grendler, Paul F. "What Zuanne Read in School: Vernacular Texts in Sixteenth Century Venetian Schools." *Sixteenth Century Journal* 13, no. 1 (1982): 41. https://doi.org/10.2307/2539916
Griffin, Clive. *The Crombergers of Seville: The History of a Printing and Merchant Dynasty*. New York: Clarendon Press, 1988.
Grmek, Mirko D., and Bernardino Fantini, eds. *Western Medical Thought from Antiquity to the Middle Ages*. Translated by Antony Shugaar. Cambridge, MA: Harvard University Press, 1998.

Gross, Charles G. *A Hole in the Head: More Tales in the History of Neuroscience*. Cambridge, MA: MIT Press, 2009.

Guerra, Francisco. "La Tradición Medieval En La Cirugía Española Del Siglo XVI." *Asclepio* 30/31 (1979–8): 359–63.

Gutiérrez Rodilla, Bertha María. "Sobre lexicografía médica del renacimiento castellano: los vocabularios de Andrés Laguna y Bartolomé Hidalgo de Agüero." *Revista de Lexicografía* 16 (December 7, 2018): 59. https://doi.org/10.17979/rlex.2010.16.0.3805

Hale, J. R. *War and Society in Renaissance Europe, 1450–1620*. New York: St. Martin's Press, 1985.

Harding, Vanessa. "Plague in Early Modern London: Chronologies, Localities, and Environments." In *Plague and the City*, edited by Lukas Engelmann, John Henderson, and Christos Lynteris, 39–68. New York: Routledge, 2019.

Harkness, Deborah E. *The Jewel House: Elizabethan London and the Scientific Revolution*. New Haven: Yale University Press, 2007.

Harper, Kristin N., Molly K. Zuckerman, Megan L. Harper, John D. Kingston, and George J. Armelagos. "The Origin and Antiquity of Syphilis Revisited: An Appraisal of Old World Pre-Columbian Evidence for Treponemal Infection." *American Journal of Physical Anthropology* 146, no. S53 (2011): 99–133. https://doi.org/10.1002/ajpa.21613

Heinrichs, Erik A. *Plague, Print, and the Reformation: The German Reform of Healing, 1473–1573*. The History of Medicine in Context. New York: Routledge, Taylor & Francis Group, 2018.

Henderson, John, Fredrika Herman Jacobs, and Jonathan K. Nelson, eds. *Representing Infirmity: Diseased Bodies in Renaissance Italy*. The Body in the City. New York: Routledge, Taylor & Francis Group, 2021.

Hernández Morejón, Antonio. *Historia bibliográfica de la medicina española (1842–1852)*. 7 vols., 1967. http://147.156.5.138/Morejon_Chinchilla/

Herrera Casado, Antonio. "Andrés Alcázar, cirujano del Renacimiento." In *Gran Enciclopedia de Castilla-La Mancha*, Vol. I. Zaragoza: Unión Aragonesa del Libro, 1982.

Herrera Dávila, Joaquín. *El Hospital del Cardenal de Sevilla y el Doctor Hidalgo de Agüero*. Sevilla: Fundación de Cultura Andaluza, 2010.

Hirsch, August. *Handbook of Geographical and Historical Pathology*. Vol. I. New Sydenham Society, 1883.

Homza, Lu Ann. "Erasmus as Hero, or Heretic? Spanish Humanism and the Valladolid Assembly of 1527." *Renaissance Quarterly* 50, no. 1 (1997): 78–118. https://doi.org/10.2307/3039329

Howick, Jeremy. "Aulus Cornelius Celsus and 'Empirical' and 'Dogmatic' Medicine." *Journal of the Royal Society of Medicine* 109, no. 11 (2016): 426–30. https://doi.org/10.1177/0141076816672397

Huguet-Termes, Teresa. "Madrid Hospitals and Welfare in the Context of the Hapsburg Empire." *Medical History. Supplement*, no. 29 (2009): 64–85.

Huizenga, Erwin. "Unintended Signatures: Middle Dutch Translations of Surgical Works." In *Science Translated: Latin and Vernacular Translations of Scientific Treatises in Medieval Europe*, edited by Michèle Goyens, Pieter de Leemans, and An Smets. Mediaevalia Lovaniensia, ser. 1, studia 40. Leuven: Leuven University Press, 2008.

Hunt, Tony. *Anglo-Norman Medicine: Roger Frugard's Chirurgia, The Practica brevis of Platearius*. Rochester NY: Boydell & Brewer, 1994.

Ieva, Antonio Di, Paolo Gaetani, Christian Matula, Camillo Sherif, Manfred Skopec, and Manfred Tschabitscher. "Berengario Da Carpi: A Pioneer in Neurotraumatology: Historical Vignette." *Journal of Neurosurgery* 114, no. 5 (2011): 1461–70. https://doi.org/10.3171/2010.10.JNS101331

Jiménez Muñoz, Juan Manuel. *Médicos y Cirujanos en "Quitaciones de Corte" (1435–1715).* Valladolid: Universidad de Valladolid, 1977.

Johns, Adrian. *The Nature of the Book: Print and Knowledge in the Making*. Chicago: University of Chicago Press, 1998.

Kagan, Richard L., and Abigail Dyer, eds. *Inquisitorial Inquiries: Brief Lives of Secret Jews and Other Heretics*. Baltimore, MD: Johns Hopkins University Press, 2011.

Kamen, Henry. *Philip of Spain*. New Haven: Yale University Press, 1997.

———. *Spain, 1469–1714: A Society of Conflict*. Third. New York: Pearson/Longman, 2005.

———. *The Spanish Inquisition: A Historical Revision*. New Haven, CT: Yale University Press, 1998.

Karplus, Heinrich, ed. *International Symposium on Society, Medicine and the Law, Jerusalem, March 1972*. New York: Elsevier Scientific Publishing Co, 1973.

Kassell, Lauren. "Casebooks in Early Modern England: Medicine, Astrology, and Written Records." *Bulletin of the History of Medicine* 88, no. 4 (2014): 595–625.

Kasten, Lloyd. "Alfonso El Sabio and the Thriteenth-Century Spanish Language." In *Emperor of Culture: Alfonso X the Learned of Castile and His Thirteenth-Century Renaissance*, edited by Robert Ignatius Burns, 33–45. Philadelphia: University of Pennsylvania Press, 1990.

Kerwin, William. *Beyond the Body: The Boundaries of Medicine and English Renaissance Drama*. Amherst: University of Massachusetts Press, 2005.

Keynes, Geoffrey, ed. *Apologie and Treatise of Ambroise Pare, Containing the Voyages Made Into Divers Places With Many of His Writings Upon Surgery*. Edited & with an Introduction by Geoffrey Keynes. The University of Chicago Press, 1952.

Kirkham, Anne, and Cordelia Warr, eds. *Wounds in the Middle Ages*. New York: Routledge, 2014.

Kirkup, John, ed. "Elective Amputation: Early Evolution to the End of the 17th Century." In *A History of Limb Amputation*, 55–67. London: Springer, 2007. https://doi.org/10.1007/978-1-84628-509-7_6

Klestinec, Cynthia. "Translating Learned Surgery." *Journal of the History of Medicine and Allied Sciences* 72, no. 1 (2017): 34–50.

———. "Vesalius among the Surgeons." *Journal of Medieval and Early Modern Studies* 48, no. 1 (January 1, 2018): 125–51. https://doi.org/10.1215/10829636-4280882

Kusukawa, Sachiko. *Picturing the Book of Nature: Image, Text, and Argument in Sixteenth-Century Human Anatomy and Medical Botany*. Chicago IL: University of Chicago Press, 2012.

Lazure, Guy. "To Dare Fame: Constructing a Cultural Elite in Sixteenth Century Seville." Ph.D., Johns Hopkins University, 2003.

Leong, Elaine. "Learning Medicine by the Book: Reading and Writing Surgical Manuals in Early Modern London." *BJHS Themes* 5 (2020): 93–110. https://doi.org/10.1017/bjt.2020.7

Leong, Elaine, and Alisha Rankin, eds. *Secrets and Knowledge in Medicine and Science, 1500–1800*. New York: Routledge, 2011.

Levin, Michael Jacob. *Agents of Empire: Spanish Ambassadors in Sixteenth-Century Italy*. Ithaca, NY: Cornell University Press, 2005.

Limbach, Saskia. "Advertising Medical Studies in Sixteenth-Century Basel: Function and Use of Academic Disputations." *Broadsheets*, 2017, 376–98. https://doi.org/10.1163/9789004340312_017

Lind, L.R., ed. "Berengario Da Carpi on Fracture of the Skull or Cranium." *Transactions of the American Philosophical Society* 80, no. 4 (1990). https://doi.org/10.2307/1006547

Littman, Robert J. "The Plague of Athens: Epidemiology and Paleopathology." *The Mount Sinai Journal of Medicine, New York* 76, no. 5 (October 2009): 456–67. https://doi.org/10.1002/msj.20137

Lloyd, G. E. R. *The Revolutions of Wisdom*. Berkeley: University of California Press, 1989.

Long, Pamela O. *Artisan/Practitioners and the Rise of the New Sciences, 1400–1600*. Corvallis: Oregon State University Press, 2011.

———. *Openness, Secrecy, Authorship: Technical Arts and the Culture of Knowledge from Antiquity to the Renaissance*. Baltimore: Johns Hopkins University Press, 2001.

López Pérez, Miguel. "Spanish Paracelsus Revisited and Decontaminated." *Azogue* 7 (2010): 339–65.

López Pérez, Miguel, and Mar Rey Bueno. "Simón de Tovar (1528–1596): redes familiares, naturaleza americana y comercio de maravillas en la Sevilla del XVI." *Dynamis: Acta Hispanica ad Medicinae Scientiarumque Historiam Illustrandam* 26 (2006): 69–91.

López Pérez, Miguel, Didier Kahn, and Mar Rey Bueno, eds. *Chymia: Science and Nature in Medieval and Early Modern Europe*. Newcastle upon Tyne, UK: Cambridge Scholars Publishing, 2010.

López Piñero, José M. "The Faculty of Medicine of Valencia." In *Universities and Science in the Early Modern Period*, edited by Mordechai Feingold and Víctor Navarro Brotons, 65–82. Archimedes, v. 12. Dordrecht: Springer, 2006.

———. "The Vesalian Movement in Sixteenth-Century Spain." *Journal of the History of Biology* 12, no. 1 (1979a): 45–81.

———. *Ciencia y técnica en la sociedad española de los siglos XVI y XVII*. Barcelona: Labor Universitaria, 1979b.

———. "El Siglo XVI." In *Historia de la medicina valenciana. Tomo I*, edited by José María López Piñero. Valencia: Vicent García Editores, 1988a.

———, ed. *Historia de la medicina valenciana. Tomo I*. Valencia: García, 1988b.

———. *La trepanación en España; clásicos neuroquirúrgicos españoles*. Madrid: Editorial Técnica Española, 1967.

———. "Nine Centuries of Cranial Surgery." *The Lancet* 2000, no. 354 (December 1, 1999): SIV35. https://doi.org/10.1016/S0140-6736(99)90378-1

———. "Paracelsus and His Work in 16th and 17th Century Spain." *Clio Medica* 8, no. 2 (1973): 113–41.

López Piñero, José María, and Francesc Bujosa Homar. "Tradición y renovación de los saberes médicos en la españa del siglo XVI." *Medicina Española* 77 (1978): 355–66.

López Piñero, José María, and Francisco Calero. *Los temas polémicos de la medicina renacentista: Las "Controversias" (1556) de Francisco Vallés*. Madrid: Consejo Superior de Investigaciones Científicas, 1988.

López Piñero, José María, and Luis García Ballester. *La obra de Andrés Alcazar sobre la trepanación*. Valencia: Cátedra e Instituto de Historia de la Medicina, 1964.

López Piñero, José María, and María Luz López Terrada. *La influencia española en la introducción en Europa de las plantas americanas (1493–1623)*. Valencia: Universitat de VALÈNCIA - C. S. I. C., 1997.

López Piñero, José María, and Jose Pardo Tomás. *La influencia de Francisco Hernández (1512–1587) en la constitución de la botánica y la materia médica modernas*. Valencia: Universitat de Valencia, 1996.

López Piñero, José, Thomas F. Glick, Víctor Navarro Brotons, and Eugenio Portela Marco. *Diccionario Histórico de La Ciencia Moderna En España*. 1a ed. 2 vols. Barcelona: Península, 1983.

López Terrada, María Luz. "Flora and the Hapsburg Crown: Clusius, Spain, and American Natural History." In *Silent Messengers: The Circulation of Material Objects of Knowledge in the Early Modern Low Countries*, edited by Sven Dupré and Christoph Lüthy. Berlin: LIT, 2011.

———. "Health Care and Poor Relief in the Crown of Aragon." In *Health Care and Poor Relief in Counter-Reformation Europe*, edited by Ole Peter Grell, Andrew Cunningham, and Jon Arrizabalaga, 177–200. New York: Routledge, 1999.

———. "Medical Pluralism in the Iberian Kingdoms: The Control of Extra-academic Practitioners in Valencia." *Medical History Supplement* 29 (2009): 7–25.
———. "Médicos, Cirujanos, Boticarios y Albéitares." In *Historia de la ciencia y de la técnica en la Corona de Castilla*, edited by Luis García Ballester, III:161–85. Valladolid: Junta de Castilla y León, Consejería de Educación y Cultura, 2002.
———. "The Control of Medical Practice under the Spanish Monarchy During the Sixteenth and Seventeenth Centuries." In *Más allá de la Leyenda Negra: España y la revolución científica = Beyond the Black Legend; Spain and the Scientific Revolution*, edited by Víctor Navarro Brotons and William Eamon, 281–94. Valencia: Univ. de València, Inst. de Historia de la Ciencia y Documentación López Piñero, 2007.
———. "The Making of Chemical Medicines in Valencia During the 16th Century: LLorenc Cocar." In *Chymia: Science and Nature in Medieval and Early Modern Europe*, edited by Miguel López Pérez, Didier Kahn, and Mar Rey Bueno, 262–78. Newcastle upon Tyne, UK: Cambridge Scholars, 2010.
López Terrada, Maria Luz, and Carmel Ferragud. "Personatges i Espais de Ciència: L'Hospital General de València En Els Seus Primers Temps." Universitat de València. Accessed March 1, 2022. https://www.uv.es/uvweb/unidad-cultura-cientifica-innovacion-catedra-divulgacion-ciencia/es/personajes-espacios-ciencia/personatges-espais-ciencia-hospital-general-valencia-els-seus-primers-temps-1286000825169/Entrevista.html?id=1285989964104
MacKay, Ruth. *Life in a Time of Pestilence: The Great Castilian Plague of 1596–1601*. New York: Cambridge University Press, 2019.
Maclean, Ian. *Logic, Signs and Nature in the Renaissance: The Case of Learned Medicine*. New York: Cambridge University Press, 2007.
———. "The Diffusion of Learned Medicine in the Sixteenth Century through the Printed Book." In *Learning and the Market Place: Essays in the History of the Early Modern Book*. Boston: Brill, 2009.
Maganto Pavón, Emilio. "Francisco Díaz." Historia de la Urología Española, n.d. http://historia.aeu.es/FranciscoDiaz.htm
———. "La Intervención Del Dr. Francisco Díaz En El Proceso Inquisitorial Contra Elena/o de Céspedes, Una Cirujana Transexual Condenada Por La Inquisición de Toledo En 1587." *Archivos Españoles de Urología* 60, no. 8 (2007): 873–86.
———. "La Operación de Talla a La Italiana Que El Licenciado Martín de Castellanos Practicó En El Escorial En 1594." *Actas Urológicas Españolas* 17 (1993): 2–7.
Malgaigne, J.-F., and Wallace B. Hamby. *Surgery and Ambroise Paré*. 1st ed. Norman: University of Oklahoma Press, 1965.
Martín Ferreira, Ana I. "El Ideal de Celso En La Cirugía Española Del s. XVI." *Medizinhistorisches Journal* 30, no. 2 (1995a): 145–65.
Martín Ferreira, Ana Isabel. *El Humanismo Médico En La Universidad de Alcalá: Siglo XVI*. Alcalá: Universidad de Alcalá, 1995b.
Martín Santos, Luis. *Barberos y cirujanos de los siglos XVI y XVII*. Valladolid: Junta de Castilla y León, Consejería de Educación y Cultura, 2000.
Martínez Ruiz, Enrique. "Felipe II, Impulsor de La Ciencia y La Técnica." In *Felipe II, la ciencia y la técnica*, edited by Enrique Martínez Ruiz, 11–14. Madrid: Actas Editorial, 1999a.
———, ed. *Felipe II, La ciencia y la técnica*. Madrid: Actas Editorial, 1999b.
Mattei, Luca. "Estudio de la Madraza de Granada a partir del registro arqueológico y de las metodologías utilizadas en la intervención del 2006." *Arqueología y Territorio*, no. 5 (2008): 181–92.
Mattern, Susan P. *The Prince of Medicine: Galen in the Roman Empire*. New York: Oxford University Press, 2013.

McCleery, Iona. "Medical Licensing in Late Medieval Portugal." In *Medicine and the Law in the Middle Ages*, edited by Wendy J. Turner and Sara M. Butler, 196–219. Medieval Law and Its Practice, volume 17. Leiden: Brill, 2014.

McVaugh, Michael. "Surgical Education in the Middle Ages." *Dynamis: Acta Hispanica ad Medicinae Scientiarumque Historiam Illustrandam* 20 (2000): 283–304.

———. "When Universities First Encountered Surgery." *Journal of the History of Medicine and Allied Sciences* 72, no. 1 (2017): 6–20.

McVaugh, Michael, and Luis García Ballester. "The Medical Faculty at Early Fourteenth-Century Lérida." In *History of Universities*, edited by Laurence Brockliss, 1–25. History of Universities 8. Oxford: Oxford Univ. Press, 1989.

McVaugh, Michael R. "Academic Medicine and the Vernacularization of Medieval Surgery: The Case of Bernat de Berriac." In *El saber i les llengües vernacles a l'època de Llull i Eiximenis: estudis ICREA sobre vernacularització*, edited by Anna Alberni, Lola Badia, Lluís Cifuentes, and Alexander Fidora. Textos i estudis de cultura catalana 170. Barcelona: Publicacions de l'Abadia de Montserrat, 2012.

———. *Medicine before the Plague: Practitioners and Their Patients in the Crown of Aragon, 1285–1345*. Cambridge Studies in the History of Medicine. Cambridge: Cambridge University Press, 2002.

———. *The Rational Surgery of the Middle Ages*. Micrologus' Library 15. Firenze: SISMEL-Edizione del Galluzzo, 2006.

Millán, Cristina Álvarez. "Graeco-Roman Case Histories and Their Influence on Medieval Islamic Clinical Accounts." *Social History of Medicine* 12, no. 1 (April 1, 1999): 19–43. https://doi.org/10.1093/shm/12.1.19

———. "The Case History in Medieval Islamic Medical Literature: Tajārib and Mujarrabāt as Source." *Medical History* 54, no. 2 (2010): 195–214. https://doi.org/10.1017/S0025727300006712

Minuzzi, Sabrina. "Printing Medical Knowledge: Vernacular Genres, Reception and Dissemination." *Nuncius* 36, no. 2 (June 23, 2021): 193–97. https://doi.org/10.1163/18253911-03602015

Montero Cartelle, Enrique. "Benito Arias Montano y Francisco Arceo: la redacción del *De recta curandorum vulnerum ratione*." *Asclepio* 64, no. 2 (2012): 417–34. https://doi.org/10.3989/asclepio.2012.v64.i2.527

Moran, Bruce T., ed. *Patronage and Institutions: Science, Technology, and Medicine at the European Court, 1500–1750*. Rochester, NY: Boydell Press, 1991.

Moreno Torres, Angela, and Mariano Pérez Albacete. "Urological Terminology in Francisco Díaz: An Example in the History of the Spanish Language." *Archivos Españoles de Urología* 56, no. 7 (2003): 739–54.

Moreno-Egea, Alfredo. "Aportaciones de los cirujanos españoles del Renacimiento." *Revista Hispanoamericana de Hernia* 4, no. 4 (October 2016): 163–72. https://doi.org/10.1016/j.rehah.2016.04.001

Morgado, Alonso. *Historia de Sevilla*. cc, 1587.

Morgan, Thomas E. "Plague or Poetry? Thucydides on the Epidemic at Athens." *Transactions of the American Philological Association* 124 (1994): 197–209. https://doi.org/10.2307/284291.

Morton, A. G. *History of Botanical Science: An Account of the Development of Botany from Ancient Times to the Present Day*. New York: Academic Press, 1981.

Muñoz Calvo, Sagrario. "El medicamento en la Medicina de Cámara de Felipe II: Protagonismo de Juan Fragoso." In *La Ciencia En El Monasterio Del Escorial*, edited by Francisco Javier Campos, 244–74. Colección Del Instituto Escurialense de Investigaciones Históricas y Artisticas, no. 3. Madrid: Ediciones Escurialenses, 1992.

Muñoz Garrido, Rafael. *Empiricos Sanitarios espanoles de los siglos XVI y XVII*. Vol. 6. Cuadernos de Historia de La Medicina Española. Monografias. Salamanca: Universidad de Salamanca, 1967.

Murphy, Hannah. *A New Order of Medicine: The Rise of Physicians in Reformation Nuremberg*. Pittsburgh: University of Pittsburgh Press, 2019.

———. "Skin and Disease in Early Modern Medicine: Jan Jessen's De Cute, et Cutaneis Affectibus (1601)." *Bulletin of the History of Medicine* 94, no. 2 (2020): 179–214. https://doi.org/10.1353/bhm.2020.0034

Nader, Helen. *The Mendoza Family in the Spanish Renaissance, 1350 to 1550*. New Brunswick, N.J: Rutgers University Press, 1979.

Navarro Brotons, Víctor, and William Eamon, eds. *Más allá de la Leyenda Negra: España y la Revolución Científica = Beyond the Black Legend: Spain and the Scientific Revolution*. Valencia: Univ. de València, Inst. de Historia de la Ciencia y Documentación López Piñero, 2007.

Newson, Linda A. *Making Medicines in Early Colonial Lima, Peru: Apothecaries, Science and Society*. Atlantic World: Europe, Africa and the Americas, 1500–1830, volume 34. Boston: Brill, 2017.

Newson, Linda A., and Susie Minchin. *From Capture to Sale: The Portuguese Slave Trade to Spanish South America in the Early Seventeenth Century*. The Atlantic World, v. 12. Leiden; Boston: Brill, 2007.

Nicaise, E., trans. and ed. *Chirurgie de maitre Henri de Mondeville, chirurgien de Philippe le Bel, roi de France, composée de 1306 à 1320*. Paris: F. Alcan, 1893.

Nummedal, Tara E. *Alchemy and Authority in the Holy Roman Empire*. Chicago: University of Chicago Press, 2007.

Nutton, Vivian. *Ancient Medicine*. New York: Routledge, 2009a.

———. "Humanist Surgery." In *The Medical Renaissance of the Sixteenth Century*, edited by A. Wear, R. K. French, and Iain M. Lonie, 75–99. New York: Cambridge University Press, 2009b.

———. "Medical Humanism, a Problematic Formulation?" *Arts et Savoirs*, no. 15. Accessed December 30, 2021. https://doi.org/10.4000/aes.3925

———. "Pieter Van Foreest: The Physician as Writer on Surgery." *Journal of the History of Medicine and Allied Sciences* 72, no. 1 (2017): 87–97.

———. "The Rise of Medical Humanism: Ferrara, 1464–1555." *Renaissance Studies* 11, no. 1 (1997): 2–19. https://doi.org/10.1111/j.1477-4658.1997.tb00008.x

Oliveros de Castro, María Teresa, and Eliseo Subiza Martin. *Felipe II: Estudio Médico-Histórico*. Publicaciones de La Universidad de Madrid: Monografías Científicas. Madrid: Aguilar, 1956.

Ollero Pina, José Antonio. *La Universidad de Sevilla en los siglos XVI y XVII*. Sevilla: Publicaciones de la Universidad de Sevilla, 1993.

O'Malley, Charles Donald. *Andreas Vesalius of Brussels, 1514–1564*. Berkeley: University of California Press, 1965.

———. "Dionisio Daza Chacon." In *Medizingeschichte in Unserer Zeit. Festgabe Fur Edith Heischkel-Artelt Und Walter Artelt Zum 65. Geburtstag.*, edited by Hans-Heinz Eulner, Gunter Mann, Gert Preiser, Rolf Winau, and Otto Winkelmann, 160–70. Stuttgart: Ferndinand Enke Verlag, 1971.

O'Malley, Charles Donald, and J. B. de C. M. Saunders. "The 'Relation' of Andreas Vesalius on the Death of Henry II of France." *Journal of the History of Medicine and Allied Sciences* 3 (1948): 197–213.

Oyola, Andrés. "Cirugía Taurina en el siglo XVI." *Toros de Lidia* (blog), September 21, 2017. http://torosdelidia.es/cirugia-taurina-en-el-siglo-xvi/

Pagel, Walter. *Paracelsus: An Introduction to Philosophical Medicine in the Era of the Renaissance.* New York: Karger Medical and Scientific Publishers, 1982.

Palma, Fermín. "El quehacer quirúrgico del doctor Andrés de León y su libro de cirugía. Baeza, 1590." *Boletín Del Instituto de Estudios Giennenses* 185 (2003): 341–54.

Palma, Jose-Alberto, and Fermin Palma. "Neurology and Don Quixote." *European Neurology* 68, no. 4 (2012): 247–57. https://doi.org/10.1159/000341338

Pardo Tomás, José. *Un lugar para la ciencia: escenarios de práctica científica en la sociedad hispana del siglo XVI.* La Orotava, Tenerife: Fundación Canaria Orotava de Historia de la Ciencia, 2006.

———. "Autores médicos en los índices inquisitoriales españoles del siglo XVI." *Dynamis: Acta Hispanica ad Medicinae Scientiarumque Historiam Illustrandam* 5–6 5 (January 1, 1985).

Park, Katharine. *Doctors and Medicine in Early Renaissance Florence.* Princeton, NJ: Princeton University Press, 1985.

———. "Medicine and Society in Medieval Europe, 500–1500." In *Medicine in Society: Historical Essays*, edited by A. Wear, 59–90. New York: Cambridge University Press, 1992.

———. "Observation in the Margins, 500–1500." In *Histories of Scientific Observation*, edited by Lorraine Daston and Elizabeth Lunbeck, 15–44. Chicago, IL: University of Chicago Press, 2011.

———. "The Criminal and the Saintly Body: Autopsy and Dissection in Renaissance Italy." *Renaissance Quarterly* 47, no. 1 (1994): 1–33. https://doi.org/10.2307/2863109.

Parker, Geoffrey. *Imprudent King: A New Life of Philip II.* New Haven: Yale University Press, 2014.

———. *Philip II.* 4th ed. Chicago: Open Court, 2002.

———. *The Military Revolution: Military Innovation and the Rise of the West, 1500–1800.* New York: Cambridge University Press, 1988.

Parshall, Karen Hunger, Michael Thomson Walton, and Bruce T. Moran, eds. *Bridging Traditions: Alchemy, Chemistry, and Paracelsian Practices in the Early Modern Era.* Early Modern Studies Series 15. Kirksville, MO: Truman State University Press, 2015.

Pérez Pastor, Cristóbal. *Bibliografía madrileña o Descripción de las obras impresas en Madrid.* Tipografía de los Huérfanos, 1907.

Pattenden, Miles, and Piers Baker-Bates, eds. *The Spanish Presence in Sixteenth-Century Italy: Images of Iberia.* New York: Ashgate Publishing, Ltd., 2015.

Pelling, Margaret. *The Common Lot: Sickness, Medical Occupations and the Urban Poor in Early Modern England.* London: Longman, 1998.

Perálvarez, José Antonio. "Francisco Díaz, Padre de La Urología." *Historias de Alcalá* (blog), Publicado el agosto 2015. https://historiasdealcala.wordpress.com/2015/08/03/francisco-diaz-padre-de-la-urologia/

Pereira, Michela. "Alchemy and the Use of Vernacular Languages in the Late Middle Ages." *Speculum* 74, no. 2 (April 1999): 336–56. https://doi.org/10.2307/2887050

Pérez Ibáñez, M. Jesús. *El humanismo médico del siglo XVI en la universidad de salamanca.* Serie Lingüística y Filología, no. 31. Valladolid: Universidad de Valladolid, Secretariado de Publicaciones e Intercambio Científico, 1998.

Pettegree, Andrew, ed. *Broadsheets: Single-Sheet Publishing in the First Age of Print.* Brill, 2017.

———. *The Book in the Renaissance.* New Haven, CT: Yale University Press, 2011.

Picatoste y Rodríguez, Felipe. *Apuntes para una biblioteca científica española del siglo XVI.* Madrid, 1891.

Plata y Marcos, Miguel de la. *Estudios biográfico-bibliográficos de la medicina militar española.* Madrid: Imp. de Manuel Álvarez, 1864.

Pomata, Gianna. “A Word of the Empirics: The Ancient Concept of Observation and Its Recovery in Early Modern Medicine.” *Annals of Science* 68, no. 1 (2011a): 1–25. https://doi.org/10.1080/00033790.2010.495039

———. “Observation Rising: Birth of an Epistemic Genre, 1500–1650.” In *Histories of Scientific Observation*, edited by Lorraine Daston and Elizabeth Lunbeck, 45–80. Chicago, IL: University of Chicago Press, 2011b.

———. “Sharing Cases: The *Observationes* in Early Modern Medicine.” *Early Science and Medicine* 15, no. 3 (2010): 193–236. https://doi.org/10.1163/157338210X493932

Porcar, Lucía Aleixandre. “Las Prácticas Quirúrgicas En Los Libros de Cirugía En Castellano Del Siglo XVII.” Tesis doctoral, Universitat de Vàlencia, 2020.

Pormann, Peter E., ed. *The Cambridge Companion to Hippocrates*. New York: Cambridge University Press, 2018.

Porter, Roy, and Mikuláš Teich, eds. *The Renaissance in National Context*. New York: Cambridge University Press, 1992.

Portuondo, María M. *Secret Science: Spanish Cosmography and the New World*. Chicago: University of Chicago Press, 2009.

———. *The Spanish Disquiet: The Biblical Natural Philosophy of Benito Arias Montano*. Chicago: The University of Chicago Press, 2019.

———. “The Study of Nature, Philosophy, and the Royal Library of San Lorenzo of the Escorial.” *Renaissance Quarterly* 63, no. 4 (2010): 1106–50. https://doi.org/10.1086/658508.

Pouchelle, Marie-Christine. *The Body and Surgery in the Middle Ages*. New Brunswick, NJ: Rutgers University Press, 1990.

Price, R. “Spanish Medicine in the Golden Age.” *Journal of the Royal Society of Medicine* 72, no. 11 (1979): 864–74.

Prieto Aguirre, Jose F. *Vida y Obra de Andres de Leon*. Vol. II, no. 5. Estudios de Historia de La Medicina Española. Salamanca: Universidad de Salamanca, 1960.

Principe, Lawrence. *The Secrets of Alchemy*. Chicago IL: University of Chicago Press, 2013.

Prioreschi, Plinio. “Skull Trauma in Egyptian and Hippocratic Medicine.” *Gesnerus* 50, no. 3–4 (1993): 167–78. https://doi.org/10.1163/22977953-0500304002

Quétel, Claude. *History of Syphilis*. Baltimore: Johns Hopkins University Press, 1992.

Rabier, Christelle. “Medicalizing the Surgical Trade, 1650–1820: Workers, Knowledge, Markets and Politics.” In *The Palgrave Handbook of the History of Surgery*, edited by Thomas Schlich, 71–94. London: Palgrave Macmillan, 2018.

Ray, Meredith K. *Daughters of Alchemy: Women and Scientific Culture in Early Modern Italy*. Cambridge, MA: Harvard University Press, 2015. https://doi.org/10.4159/9780674425873

Reeds, Karen. *Botany in Medieval and Renaissance Universities*. Harvard Dissertations in the History of Science. New York: Garland, 1991.

Rekers, Ben. *Benito Arias Montano (1527–1598)*. Studies of the Warburg Institute 33. Leiden: E.J. Brill, 1972.

Rey Bueno, Mar, and María Esther Alegre Pérez. “Los Destiladores de Su Majestad. Destilación, espagiria y paracelsismo en la corte de Felipe II.” *Dynamis: Acta Hispanica ad Medicinae Scientiarumque Historiam Illustrandam* 21 (2001): 323–50.

Richardson, Brian. *Print Culture in Renaissance Italy: The Editor and the Vernacular Text, 1470–1600*. First Edition. Cambridge England; New York: Cambridge University Press, 1994.

Riera, Juan. “La Obra de Francisco Arceo.” *Cuadernos de Historia de La Medicina Espanola* 3 (1964): 96–8.

———. *Vida y Obra de Luis Mercado*. Ediciones Del Seminario e Historia de La Medicina Española. Salamanca: Universidad de Salamanca, 1968.

Rissech, Carme, Charlotte Roberts, Xavier Tomás-Batlle, Xavier Tomás-Gimeno, Benjamin Fuller, Pedro Luis Fernandez, and Miguel Botella. "A Roman Skeleton with Possible Treponematosis in the North-East of the Iberian Peninsula: A Morphological and Radiological Study: Possible Treponematosis in Late Roman Iberia?" *International Journal of Osteoarchaeology* 23, no. 6 (November 2013): 651–63. https://doi.org/10.1002/oa.1293

Rodrigues, Isilda, and Carlos Fiolhais. "La censura inquisitorial en las centurias de Amatus Lusitanus." *Asclepio: Revista de Historia de La Medicina y de La Ciencia* 70, no. 2 (December 20, 2018): 229. https://doi.org/10.3989/asclepio.2018.13

Rodríguez-Sala, María Luisa. *Los cirujanos de hospitales de la Nueva España (siglos XVI y XVII): miembros de un estamento profesional o de una comunidad científica?* Mexico City: Universidad Nacional Autónoma de México, 2005.

Rodríguez Salgado, M. J. "«Una perfecta princesa». Casa y vida de la reina Isabel de Valois (1559–1568). Primera Parte." *Cuadernos de Historia Moderna*, 2003, 39–96.

Rojo Vega. "Antonio Pérez y el doctor portugués. De la cirugía a la peste." *Revista Espanola de Investigaciones Quirurgicas* XVII, no. 1 (2014): 49–55.

———. *Enfermos y sanadores en la Castilla del siglo XVI*. Historia y sociedad 34. Valladolid: Universidad de Valladolid, 1993.

San Román Gómez, Ricardo. "La Obra Quirúrgica de Juan Calvo." *A Medicina Contemporânea* 79 (1961): 75–104.

Sánchez Capelot, Francisco. *La Obra Quirúgica de Francisco Díaz*. Publicaciones Del Seminario de Historia de La Medicina de La Universidad de Salamanca. Serie A, Estudios. Salamanca: Seminario de Historia de la Medicina de la Universidad de Salamanca, 1959.

———. *La obra quirúgica de Juan Fragoso*. Publicaciones del Seminario de Historia de la Medicina de la Universidad de Salamanca. Serie A, Estudios. Salamanca: Seminario de Historia de la Medicina de la Universidad de Salamanca, 1957.

Sánchez-Martín, F. M., A. M. Hostalot, J. M. Santillana, O. Angerri, F. Millán, and H. Villavicencio. "Extraction of a Bladder Stone in a Child as Described by the Renaissance Physician Cristóbal Méndez." *Actas Urologicas Espanolas* 38, no. 7 (September 2014): 476–82. https://doi.org/10.1016/j.acuro.2014.02.002

Savage-Smith, E. "The Practice of Surgery in Islamic Lands: Myth and Reality." *Social History of Medicine* 13, no. 2 (2000): 307–21. https://doi.org/10.1093/shm/13.2.307

Savoia, Paolo. *Gaspare Tagliacozzi and Early Modern Surgery: Faces, Men, and Pain*. New York: Routledge, 2019a.

———. "Skills, Knowledge, and Status: The Career of an Early Modern Italian Surgeon." *Bulletin of the History of Medicine* 93, no. 1 (2019b): 27–54. https://doi.org/10.1353/bhm.2019.0001

———. "Suffering through It: Visual and Textual Representations of Bodies in Surgery in the Wake of Lepanto (1571)." In *Representing Infirmity: Diseased Bodies in Renaissance Italy*, edited by John Henderson, Fredrika Herman Jacobs, and Jonathan K. Nelson, 141–66. The Body in the City. New York: Routledge, Taylor & Francis Group, 2021.

Schlich, Thomas, ed. *The Palgrave Handbook of the History of Surgery*. London: Palgrave Macmillan, 2018.

Scribner, Bob. "Is a History of Popular Culture Possible?" *History of European Ideas* 10, no. 2 (January 1, 1989): 175–91. https://doi.org/10.1016/0191-6599(89)90067-3

Shotwell, R. Allen. "The Great Pox and the Surgeon's Role in the Sixteenth Century." *Journal of the History of Medicine and Allied Sciences* 72, no. 1 (2017): 21–33.

Siena, Kevin, ed. *Sins of the Flesh: Responding to Sexual Disease in Early Modern Europe*. Toronto: Centre for Reformation and Renaissance Studies, 2005.

Simili, Alessandro. "The Beginnings of Forensic Medicine in Bologna." In *International Symposium on Society, Medicine and the Law, Jerusalem, March 1972*, 91–100. New York: Elsevier Scientific Publishing Co, 1973.

Singer, Charles. "The Early Treatment of Gunshot Wounds." *The Quarterly Review* 226, no. 449 (1916): 452–69.

Siraisi, Nancy G. "How to Write a Latin Book on Surgery: Organizing Principles and Authorial Devices in Guglielmo Da Saliceto and Dino Del Garbo." In *Practical Medicine from Salerno to the Black Death*, edited by Luis García Ballester, Roger French, Jon Arrizabalaga, and Andrew Cunningham, 88–109. New York: Cambridge University Press, 1994.

———. *Medieval & Early Renaissance Medicine: An Introduction to Knowledge and Practice.* Chicago: University of Chicago Press, 1990.

———. *Taddeo Alderotti and His Pupils: Two Generations of Italian Medical Learning.* Princeton: Princeton University Press, 2019. https://doi.org/10.1515/9780691198163

———. "The Changing Fortunes of a Traditional Text: Goals and Strategies in Sixteenth-Century Latin Editions of the Canon of Avicenna." In *The Medical Renaissance of the Sixteenth Century*, edited by A. Wear, R. K. French, and Iain M. Lonie, 16–41. New York: Cambridge University Press, 2009.

Skaarup, Bjørn Okholm. *Anatomy and Anatomists in Early Modern Spain.* History of Medicine in Context. Burlington, VT: Ashgate, 2015.

Slack, Paul. "Mirrors of Health and Treasures of Poor Men: The Uses of Vernacular Medical Literature of Tudor England." In *Health, Medicine and Mortality in the Sixteenth Century*, edited by Webster, Charles, 237–73. Cambridge University Press, 1979.

Smith, Pamela H. *The Business of Alchemy: Science and Culture in the Holy Roman Empire.* Princeton, NJ: Princeton University Press, 1994.

Smith, Pamela H., and Paula Findlen, eds. *Merchants and Marvels: Commerce, Science, and Art in Early Modern Europe.* New York: Routledge, 2002.

Smith, Pamela H., Amy R. W. Meyers, and Harold J. Cook, eds. *Ways of Making and Knowing: The Material Culture of Empirical Knowledge.* Ann Arbor: University of Michigan Press, 2014.

Solano Alonso, Jairo. *Salud, cultura y sociedad: Cartagena de Índias, siglos XVI y XVII.* Barranquilla: Universidad del Atlántico, 1998.

Solomon, Michael Ray. "Translating Disease: The Vernacular Medical Treatise in the Late Medieval Kingdom of Aragon," 1994. https://buleria.unileon.es/handle/10612/6360

Solomon, Michael. *Fictions of Well-Being: Sickly Readers and Vernacular Medical Writing in Late Medieval and Early Modern Spain.* Philadelphia: University of Pennsylvania Press, 2010.

Somolinos d'Ardois, Germán. *Vida y Obra de Francisco Hernández: Precedida de España y Nueva España En La Época de Felipe II.* 1st ed. México: Universidad Nacional de México, 1960.

Soriano de la Rosa, Concepcion. *La obra quirúrgica de Dionisio Daza Chacón.* Publicaciones del Seminario de Historia de la Medicina de la Universidad de Salamanca, Serie A: Estudios,; t. 2, no. 1; Salamanca, 1958.

Staden, Heinrich von. *Herophilus: The Art of Medicine in Early Alexandria.* New York: Cambridge University Press, 1989.

Stein, Claudia. *Negotiating the French Pox in Early Modern Germany.* The History of Medicine in Context. Burlington, VT: Ashgate, 2009.

Stolberg, Michael. *Uroscopy in Early Modern Europe.* Translated by Logan Kennedy and Leonhard Unglaub. The History of Medicine in Context. Burlington, VT: Ashgate, 2015.

Stone, Howard. "The French Language in Renaissance Medicine." *Bibliothèque d'Humanisme et Renaissance* 15, no. 3 (1953): 315–46.

Taape, Tillmann. "Common Medicine for the Common Man: Picturing the 'Striped Layman' in Early Vernacular Print." *Renaissance Quarterly* 74, no. 1 (2021): 1–58. https://doi.org/10.1017/rqx.2020.315

Taavitsainen, Irma, and Päivi Pahta, eds. *Medical and Scientific Writing in Late Medieval English*. Studies in English Language. New York: Cambridge University Press, 2004a.

———. "Vernacularisation of Scientific and Medical Writing in Its Sociohistorical Context." In *Medical and Scientific Writing in Late Medieval English*, edited by Irma Taavitsainen and Päivi Pahta, 1–19. Studies in English Language. New York: Cambridge University Press, 2004b.

Tausiet, Maria. "Fool's Silver: Alchemy and Fraud in Sixteenth-Century Spain." In *Chymia: Science and Nature in Medieval and Early Modern Europe*, edited by Miguel López Pérez, Didier Kahn, and Mar Rey Bueno, 18. Newcastle upon Tyne, UK: Cambridge Scholars Publishing, 2010.

Taylor, J.S. "United States Naval Medical Bulletin. v. 15, 1921." *United States Naval Medical Bulletin*. v. 15, 1921 XV, no. 3 (1921): 561–626.

Thomas, Duncan P. "Thomas Vicary and the Anatomie of Mans Body." *Medical History* 50, no. 02 (2006): 235–46. https://doi.org/10.1017/S0025727300009765

Torre, Esteban. "Las 'conclusiones' del doctor Estrada de Madrid, contra los 'Avisos Particulares' del doctor Hidalgo de Aguero, Sevillano." *Asclepio* 30/31 (79 1978): 389–401.

Torre Revello, Jose. *El libro, la imprenta y el periodismo en América durante la dominación española*. no. 74. Buenos Aires: Publicaciones del Instituto de Investigaciones Historicas, 1940.

Tracy, Larissa, and Kelly DeVries, eds. *Wounds and Wound Repair in Medieval Culture*. Explorations in Medieval Culture, Vol. 1. Boston: Brill, 2015.

Ungerer, Gustav. "George Baker: Translator of Aparicio de Zubia's Pamphlet on the 'Oleum Magistrale.'" *Medical History* 30, no. 02 (1986): 203–11. https://doi.org/10.1017/S0025727300045397

Vallejo, José Ramón, Marina Mesa, and José M Cobos-Bueno. "Francisco Arceo de Fregenal and the Treatment of Clubfoot up to the Sixteenth Century." *Acta Medico-Historica Adriatica* 16, no. 1 (2018): 19–48. https://doi.org/10.31952/amha.16.1.1

Van Hee, Robert. "The Evolution of Surgery in the Low Countries during the Sixteenth Century." *Sartoniana/University of Ghent Sarton Chair of the History of Sciences* 15 (2002): 97–153.

Van Scoy, Herbert Allen, and Ivy A. Corfis. *A Dictionary of Old Spanish Terms Defined in the Works of Alfonso X*. Madison, WI: Hispanic Seminary of Medieval Studies, 1986.

van't Land, Karine. "'Because My Son Does Not Read Latin' Rhetoric, Competition and Education in Middle Dutch Surgical Handbooks'." *Studies in Ancient Medicine* 35 (2010): 443–59.

———. "The Solution of Continuous Things." In *Wounds in the Middle Ages*, edited by Anne Kirkham and Cordelia Warr. New York: Routledge, 2014.

Varey, Simon, Rafael Chabrán, and Dora B. Weiner, eds. *Searching for the Secrets of Nature: The Life and Works of Dr. Francisco Hernández*. Stanford, CA: Stanford University Press, 2000.

Vázquez Medina, D. Antonio José. "Sevillana Cirugía, 1550–1650. Escuelas Quirúrgicas de Sevilla Siglo XVI." Ph.D., Universidad de Sevilla, 2002.

Vekerdy, Lilla. "Paracelsus's Great Wound Surgery." In *Textual Healing: Essays on Medieval and Early Modern Medicine*, edited by Elizabeth Lane Furdell, 77–91. Boston: Brill, 2005.

Villalba y Guitarte, Joaquín de. *Epidemiología española o Historia cronológica de las pestes, contagios, epidemias y epizootias que han acaecido en España desde la venida de las cartagineses hasta el año 1801: con noticia de algunas otras enfermedades que han sufrido los españoles en otros reynos, y de los autores nacionales que han escrito sobre esta materia…* Madrid, 1802.

Villalon, Andrew. "The 1562 Head Injury of Don Carlos: A Conflict of Medicine and Religion in Sixteenth-Century Spain." *Mediterranean Studies* 22, no. 2 (2014): 95–134.

Villalon, L. J. Andrew. "Putting Don Carlos Together Again: Treatment of a Head Injury in Sixteenth- Century Spain." *Sixteenth Century Journal* 26, no. 2 (1995): 347–65.

Volk, Peter, and Hans Jurgen Warlo. "The Role of Medical Experts in Court Proceedings in the Medieval Town." In *International Symposium on Society, Medicine and the Law, Jerusalem, March 1972*, 101–16. New York: Elsevier Scientific Publishing Co, 1973.

Walker, Don, Natasha Powers, Brian Connell, and Rebecca Redfern. "Evidence of Skeletal Treponematosis from the Medieval Burial Ground of St. Mary Spital, London, and Implications for the Origins of the Disease in Europe: Skeletal Treponematosis from St. Mary Spital." *American Journal of Physical Anthropology* 156, no. 1 (2015): 90–101. https://doi.org/10.1002/ajpa.22630

Wallis, Faith. "Pre-Modern Surgery: Wounds, Words, and the Paradox of 'Tradition.'" In *The Palgrave Handbook of the History of Surgery*, edited by Thomas Schlich, 49–70. London: Palgrave Macmillan, 2018.

Walsby, Malcolm. "Cheap Print and the Academic Market: The Printing of Dissertations in Sixteenth-Century Louvain." In *Broadsheets: Single-Sheet Publishing in the First Age of Print*, edited by Andrew Pettegree. Brill, 2017.

Wear, A. *Knowledge and Practice in Early Modern English Medicine, 1550–1680*. New York: Cambridge University Press, 2000.

———, ed. *Medicine in Society: Historical Essays*. New York: Cambridge University Press, 1992.

Wear, A., R. K. French, and Iain M. Lonie, eds. *The Medical Renaissance of the Sixteenth Century*. New York: Cambridge University Press, 2009.

Webster, Charles, ed. *Health, Medicine and Mortality in the Sixteenth Century*. New York: 1979.

Wilkinson, Alexander S., ed. *Iberian Books/Libros ibéricos (IB): Books Published in Spanish or Portuguese or on the Iberian Peninsula before 1601/Libros publicados en español o portugués o en la Península Ibérica antes de 1601*. Boston: Brill, 2010.

Wilkinson, Alexander Samuel, and Alejandra Ulla Lorenzo, eds. *Iberian Books Volumes II & III/Libros Ibéricos Volúmenes II y III (2 vols): Books published in Spain, Portugal and the New World or elsewhere in Spanish or Portuguese between 1601 and 1650/Libros publicados en España, Portugal y el Nuevo Mundo o impresos en otros lugares en español o portugués entre 1601 y 1650*. Boston: Brill, 2015.

Wilkinson, Alexander S., Alejandra Ulla Lorenzo, and Alba de la Cruz. "A Survey of Printed Spanish Broadsheets, 1472–1700." In *Broadsheets: Single-Sheet Publishing in the First Age of Print*, 60: 55–75. Library of the Written Word. Brill, 2017.

Wilson-Lee, Edward. *The Catalogue of Shipwrecked Books: Christopher Columbus, His Son, and the Quest to Build the World's Greatest Library*. New York: Simon and Schuster, 2019.

Witt, Mathias. "Surgery." In *The Cambridge Companion to Hippocrates*, edited by Peter E. Pormann, 217–45. New York: Cambridge University Press, 2018.

Worth-Stylianou, Valerie. "Concurrent Publication of Medical Works in Neo-Latin and French in Early Modern France." *Canadian Review of Comparative Literature/Revue Canadienne de Littérature Comparée* 41, no. 4 (2014): 456–76. https://doi.org/10.1353/crc.2014.0040

Zimmerman, Leo M., and Ilza Veith. *Great Ideas in the History of Surgery*. 2d rev. ed. New York: Dover Publications, 1967.

Zinsser, Hans. *Rats, Lice, & History: Being a Study in Biography, Which, after Twelve Preliminary Chapters Indispensable for the Preparation of the Lay Reader, Deals with the Life History of Typhus Fever …* Boston: Little, Brown and Company, 1963.

INDEX

Pages followed by n refers notes.

Albucasis (al-Zahrawi) 14, 17, 57, 86
Alcalá de Henares 67, 90; University of 16, 21–2, 31, 35, 36, 41, 42, 43, 45, 126, 128, 129
Alcázar, Andrés 7, 22, 32, 33, 40, 41, 47, 48, 59, 60, 80, 85, 87, 91–3, 111, 114, 115, 125
alchemy 77, 78
algebrista *see* bones
anatomy 2, 3, 8, 13, 15, 16, 19, 21, 32, 39, 44, 45, 57, 62, 72, 75, 77, 78, 82, 85, 100, 106, 123, 128, 130
antidotary 48, 63, 101, 111, 114, 115, 126, 127, 129
Aparicio de Zubia 35, 76
apostemas 62, 72, 128, 131
Aragon, Crown of 5, 14, 15, 18–22, 31, 44, 66; Kingdom of 21, 22, 121
Arce, Alonso de 76
Arceo, Francisco 7, 17, 32, 33, 40–2, 47–9, 58, 60, 63, 66, 79, 80, 82, 87, 90, 91, 111, 114, 126; Balsamo de 41, 126
Argellata, Pietro 79
Armada 38, 39, 130
Avicenna (Ibn Sina) 14, 16, 17, 48, 57, 78, 79, 84, 86, 93, 104

Badajoz 40, 41, 126
Barcelona 18, 122
Barrios, Juan de 85, 130
bladder stones 76, 101
Bologna: teaching of surgery in 15, 17, 110; University of 14, 22, 110
bones 86, 115; bonesetters (*algebristas*) 20, 24, 35, 63, 76; broken 24, 35, 76, 82, 101
Borgognoni, Teodorico 15, 57, 59, 82
Boschi, Ippolito 109
Botallo, Leonardo 109
botany 2, 35, 42, 44, 45, 77, 78, 129; *see also* materia medica
Brassavola, Antonio Musa 17, 77
Brunschwig, Hieronymus 58, 108
Burgos 18, 36, 61, 72, 128

Calvo, Juan 7, 8, 15, 18, 23, 30–3, 40, 44, 46–8, 62, 66, 76, 85, 100, 101, 111, 114–5, 126–7, 130
da Carpi, Berengario 2, 17, 47, 48, 49, 85, 88, 89, 93, 108, 109
case studies 4, 9, 30, 41, 49, 66, 78, 79, 80, 93, 122
Castañeda, Juan de 43, 77
Castile, Kingdom of 5, 14, 17–22, 31, 41, 44, 47, 60, 61, 66, 113, 121
Castilian: language 7, 9, 13, 15, 17, 32, 42, 46, 58–62, 66, 82, 84, 85, 105; universities 21, 121, 123
Catalan language 7, 60, 105
Catalonia 5, 21, 22, 121
cataracts 24, 57, 76, 101
Celsus 14, 16, 17, 48, 57, 66, 76, 79, 88, 93
Charles V 2, 7, 18, 38, 107, 130; education and regulation of medical practitioners 20–1, 121; patronage of medical practitioners 2, 33–5, 37, 76, 91, 104, 110, 127

Chauliac, Guy de 2, 15, 46, 48, 56, 58, 61, 82, 86, 93
Clowes, William 109
Clusius, Carolus (Charles de l'Écluse) 30, 42, 43, 77, 78
Coimbra 15, 22, 43
Collado, Luis 2, 21, 44, 45, 47, 127, 128
Council of Castile 22, 47, 113
Cuadra, Alonso 129
Cueva, Juan de la 43, 129

Daza Chacón, Dionisio 7, 8, 18, 30, 31–4, 36, 37–9, 44, 48, 49, 56, 62, 66, 67, 74, 76, 89–90, 100, 106, 108, 109–10, 112, 127–28
della Croce, Giovanni Andrea 58, 92
Díaz, Alfonso 35, 103, 104
Díaz, Diego 76
Díaz, Francisco 3, 7, 8, 18, 24, 32, 33, 35–7, 45, 48, 49, 62, 63, 66, 67, 72, 74, 76, 78, 80, 85, 102–07, 128
Dioscorides 77
dislocaciones/dislocations 3, 46, 57, 62, 76, 129, 131; *see also* wounds
Don Juan de Austria 38, 39, 127, 130, 131
dropsy 57
Duke of Alba 38, 89, 130, 131

empiricism 4, 8, 9, 37, 44, 59, 67, 72, 74–7, 83
empirics 19, 35, 37, 59, 63, 75, 76, 80, 84, 86, 87, 101–04, 114, 122
epidemic disease 3, 34, 36, 101, 110–16, 124; *see also* plague; typhus; morbo gálico
El Escorial 33, 35, 38, 42, 130
Eustachi, Bartolomeo 49

Falloppio, Gabriele 2, 48, 49
Fernando and Isabel 5, 20, 37, 121
Ferri, Alfonso 109
Fioravanti, Leonardo 35, 49, 109
Florentino, Nicolo (Niccolò Falcucci) 57
forensic medicine *see* legal medicine
fracturas/fractures 3, 14, 16, 32, 44, 46, 57, 62, 76, 79, 82, 84, 86, 88, 90, 91, 93, 129, 131; *see also* wounds
Fragoso, Juan 3, 7, 8, 9, 13, 30–8, 41, 43, 47–9, 58, 62, 63, 64, 66, 67, 74, 76, 78–80, 82–6, 91, 105–07, 111, 114, 115, 122, 123, 129
Franco, Francisco 43
Franco, Pierre 33
French Disease *see* morbo gálico
Frisius, Gemma 42

Gago de Vadilla, Pedro 43, 86
Gale, Thomas 109
Galen 13, 16, 17, 47, 48, 57, 66, 67, 73, 74, 75, 76, 81, 84, 87, 88, 93, 102, 104
Gesner, Conrad 49, 75
Granada 5, 15, 37, 38, 111, 130
Great Pox *see* morbo gálico
Guadalupe *see* hospitals

Haly Abbas (al-Majusi) 57
Hapsburg-Valois Wars 33, 37, 125
Hernández, Francisco 17, 35, 41, 43, 51, 54, 107, 129
hernia 24, 35, 57, 63, 76, 101, 128
Hidalgo de Aguero, Bartolomé 7, 8, 9, 18, 32, 33, 36, 38–41, 43–5, 47–9, 57–8, 62–7, 72–4, 76, 79–86, 88, 91, 93, 100, 111–13, 115, 123, 126, 129, 30
Hierro, Alonso 79
Hippocrates 13, 16, 17, 23, 47, 48, 62, 63, 66, 76, 79, 82, 84, 87, 129, 131
hospitals 4, 17–9, 31, 36, 39, 40, 112; Hospital del Cardenal (San Hermenegildo) in Seville 38, 40, 43–4, 64, 73, 82, 85, 129, 130; Hospital de la Corte in Valladolid 18, 36, 37, 127, 130; Reales Hospitales de Santa María de Guadalupe 17, 41, 126; Valencia 31, 38, 130; Zaragoza 19, 31, 38, 130
humanism 5, 7, 16–7, 72; medical 16, 119n43

Ibn Sina *see* Avicenna
Index of Forbidden Books 22, 49, 74

Jimeno, Pedro 2, 21, 45, 128

Laguna, Andrés 47, 49, 102, 106, 107
Lanfranc of Milan 2, 15, 48, 56, 61, 86
Latin texts 2, 5, 13, 14, 15, 24, 32, 35, 40, 42, 57, 58, 60, 82, 84, 91, 113, 122, 126
laudable pus 81
legal medicine 10, 13, 57, 67, 80, 105–7, 129; cause of death 10, 13, 80, 105; fertility 10, 13, 106; paternity 10
de León, Andrés 8, 31, 32, 33, 37–9, 63, 67, 76, 100, 101, 111, 113, 114, 123, 130–31
Leoniceno, Niccolò 16, 17, 115
Lérida 15, 21
llagas (heridas nuevas/new wounds) 62, 126, 127; *see also* wounds
Longoburgo, Bruno 15, 56

López de León, Pedro 43, 86, 130
Lusitano, Amato (João Rodrigues de Castelo Branco) 47, 49

Madrid 18, 21, 25, 31, 33, 34, 35, 36, 42, 43, 64, 67, 83, 90, 105, 128–30
Maggi, Bartolomeo 79, 109, 110
al-Majusi *see* Haly Abbas
materia medica 1, 8, 21, 32, 33, 35, 38, 41, 43, 83, 107
Mattioli, Pietro Andrea 49, 77
médico y cirujano 3, 7, 9, 23–5, 38, 64, 111, 112, 121
medieval surgeons/surgery 7, 9, 13–7, 19, 30, 44, 46, 48, 56–9, 61, 66, 67, 74, 78, 81–2, 84, 87, 93, 101, 108
Mercado, Luis 35, 113, 115
Monardes 38, 42, 43, 58, 77, 107, 111, 112, 130
Mondeville, Henri de 15, 19, 57, 61, 82
Mondino de Luzzi 16
Montpellier, University of 14, 15, 44, 78, 127
morbo gálico (French disease) 10, 18, 33, 39–40, 60, 67, 83, 101, 104, 110–11, 113–15, 125–26, 130

Naples 21, 22, 113–15
Navarre 5, 21, 22, 121
Nebrija, Antonio 7, 17
networks, intellectual 8, 9, 30–1, 35, 46–50; Seville 35, 38, 41–4, 83; Valencia 44–6
neurosurgery *see* trepanation

ointment 44, 48, 81, 90, 111; *see also* balsam; salve
Ortelius, Abraham 42

Padua 2, 15, 16, 86
Paracelsus 49, 74–5, 77, 106, 108
Paré, Ambroise 1, 3, 33, 34, 49, 59, 63, 89, 93, 106, 107, 108, 109, 110, 126, 128
Paris 14, 15, 19, 66, 89
Paul of Aegina 16, 17, 66, 78
Pérez, Antonio 8, 31, 32, 33, 37–9, 66, 67, 111, 113, 122, 131
Philip II 7, 18; education and regulation of surgeons 19, 21–3, 121–3; patronage of medical practitioners 33–9, 41–3, 76, 77, 89–90, 101–02, 104, 113; and Protomedicato 17, 20, 43, 113
plague: hospitals 18; treatises 39, 40, 43, 58, 60, 66, 111–3, 125; *see also* epidemic disease

Plantin, Christophe 42, 43, 60, 126
Pliny 76, 77
Portugal 15, 21, 34, 38, 39, 43, 49, 61, 114, 121, 127, 130
printing/publishing 1–3, 5, 8, 9, 10, 13, 16, 22, 25, 31, 35, 36, 40, 42, 49, 50, 57, 60–7, 72, 78, 82, 85, 88, 106, 109, 111, 114, 122–24; broadsheets 47, 64–5, 82–4, 86; images 58–60, 122; surgical texts 3, 7–10, 13, 25, 35–7, 41, 46–50, 59, 62–7, 82–3, 85
Protestantism 22, 75
Protomedicato 20–1, 23, 34, 35, 56, 83, 113, 121, 123, 127, 130
Protomédico 17, 19, 21, 31, 35, 38, 43, 102, 113

al-Rāzī *see* Rhazes
remedies 23, 75, 102, 107, 114, 115; alchemical 77; compound remedies 48, 63, 74, 76, 77, 80, 101, 115; medical simples, 13, 16, 21, 35, 44, 63; proprietary compounds 41, 76, 109; *see also* antidotary; materia medica
rete mirabile 82, 89, 97n53
Rhazes (al-Rāzī) 14, 57
Rome 22, 35, 49, 104
Rota, Giovanni Francesco 109

Salamanca, University of 7, 14, 15, 17, 21, 22, 31, 40, 43, 49, 59, 125, 127
Saliceto, William of 2, 15, 57, 86
salve 44, 77; *see also* balsam; ointment
Sanchez de Oropesa, Francisco 43, 105, 112
scabies 57, 101, 114
Seville: city of 9, 18, 31, 35, 36, 38, 40–4, 61, 64, 67, 73, 77, 82–3, 85, 105, 111–3, 122, 126, 129, 130; University of 14, 31, 38, 43, 64; *see also* networks; hospitals
Somovilla, Diego de 76
Somovilla, Francisco de 76
Sosa Sotomayor, Juan de 43, 85, 130
surgeons: Latinate/*latino* 7, 9, 23, 24, 62; military 33, 37–9, 50, 107–110, 122, 127, 130; private 31, 33, 40, 41, 50, 60, 122; *romancista* 24, 59, 62, 123; royal 18, 30, 33–9, 83–5, 89, 90, 91, 102, 104, 122, 127, 128, 129; teaching 39–46, 64, 83
syphilis *see* morbo gálico

Tovar, Simon de 41–3, 77, 107
translation: Arabic to Latin 14, 16, 57, 101; Latin to vernacular 5, 7, 13, 25, 46, 49,

58–62, 84, 88, 108; between vernacular languages 25, 36; vernacular to Latin 43, 62, 74; *see also* vernacular
trepan 9, 40, 60, 84, 88, 90–2, 125
trepanation 9, 40, 44, 67, 73, 80–1, 84, 86–92, 123, 125; Don Carlos and 37, 89–90; Henry II and 37, 89–90
trephine/trephination *see* trepan/trepanation

úlceras (llagas viejas/old wounds) 62
urology 10, 24, 33, 36–7, 40, 57, 80, 85, 101–6, 128

Valencia (city) 9, 15, 18, 20–1, 31, 38, 40, 42, 44–5, 67, 122, 127; Colegio de Barberos y Cirujanos 19; Estudi de Cirugía 15, 21, 44; Kingdom of 5, 22, 121; University of 2, 7, 16, 19, 21, 40, 45, 121, 127; *see also* networks; intellectual
Valladolid 18, 36, 37, 67, 104, 119, 122, 127, 128; University of 14, 21, 22, 31, 113
Valles, Francisco 13, 35, 45, 47, 49, 102, 106, 115
Vega, Cristóbal de 35, 47, 90
vernacular (*romance*) 3, 5, 32, 41, 56, 58–62, 64, 65, 67, 84, 88, 91, 102, 121–3; texts 3, 7, 9, 23, 24, 35, 38, 40, 57, 58–62, 65, 66, 84, 113, 122, 123, 124, 131; *see also* translation
Vesalius 2, 13, 16, 21, 33, 37, 44, 47, 48, 89–90
vía común 44, 73, 81, 86; *see also* wounds
vía particular 43, 44, 58, 72, 80, 81, 83, 85–6, 129–30; *see also* wounds
Vicary, Thomas 33, 59
da Vigo, Giovanni 1, 33, 47, 49, 58, 85, 93, 106, 108, 115

wounds: gunpowder 10, 34, 80, 101, 107–110, 128; head/cranial 14, 33, 37, 40, 44, 57, 60, 63, 66, 73, 79, 81, 84, 86–93, 125, 126, 130; treatment of 9, 36, 43, 57–8, 64, 67, 72, 73, 78–80; wet versus dry healing 9, 81–6, 123; *see also* apostemas; fracturas; llagas; úlceras

al-Zahrawi *see* Albucasis
Zamorano, Rodrigo 43
Zamudio de Alfaro 43, 113
Zaragoza 18–20, 31, 38, 44, 67, 127; Colegio de Médicos y Cirujanos 19–20

For Product Safety Concerns and Information please contact our EU
representative GPSR@taylorandfrancis.com
Taylor & Francis Verlag GmbH, Kaufingerstraße 24, 80331 München, Germany

www.ingramcontent.com/pod-product-compliance
Ingram Content Group UK Ltd.
Pitfield, Milton Keynes, MK11 3LW, UK
UKHW021307260926
475702UK00048B/793
9781032270401